Advances in Anatomy
Embryology and Cell Biology

Vol. 80

W0050523

Editors
F. Beck, Leicester W. Hild, Galveston
J. van Limborgh, Amsterdam R. Ortmann, Köln
J.E. Pauly, Little Rock T.H. Schiebler, Würzburg

Jürgen Koebke

A Biomechanical and Morphological Analysis of Human Hand Joints

With 50 Figures

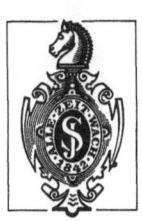

Springer-Verlag
Berlin Heidelberg New York Tokyo 1983

Priv.-Doz. Dr. Jürgen Koebke
Institute of Anatomy
University of Kiel
Olshausenstr. 40–60
D-2300 Kiel
Federal Republic of Germany

Revised version of the *Habilitation* thesis submitted to the
Medical Faculty of the Christian Albrecht University of Kiel,
1981

Library of Congress Cataloging in Publication Data
Koebke, Jürgen, 1945 – A biomechanical and morphological analysis of
human hand joints.
(Advances in anatomy, embryology, and cell biology; v. 80)
Revision of the author's Habilitationsschrift – – Christian Albrecht
University of Kiel, 1981. Bibliography: p. Includes index. 1. Hand––
Anatomy. 2. Human mechanics. 3. Joints. I. Title. II. Series. [DNLM:
1. Biomechanics. 2. Finger joint – – Anatomy and histology. 3. Wrist
joint – – Anatomy and histology. Wl AD433K v. 80/WE 830 K77b]
QL801. E67 vol. 80 574.4s [611'.717] 83-4727 [QM548]

ISBN-13: 978-3-540-12438-2   e-ISBN-13: 978-3-642-69119-5
DOI: 10.107/978-3-642-69119-5

Composition: Schreibsatz Service Weihrauch, Würzburg

2121/3321-543210

Contents

1 General Introduction

Functional morphology seeks to establish the relationship between form and function: the description of anatomic phenomena is used as a basis for defining functional factors which themselves, long term, affect the development of the form. This kind of basic study is essential for our understanding of quadruped and human motion and has been discussed by Pauwels (1948, 1955, 1960) and Kummer (1956, 1959, 1962, 1978). Biomechanical analysis of human upper and lower limb joints has resulted in causal therapy in cases of joint disease (Pauwels 1935, 1961, 1976; Maquet 1976).

Studies of the functional strain on the shoulder joint socket and the elbow joint have been carried out by Pauwels (1955, 1959, 1963) and Tillmann (1971, 1978). Joints of the human hand and wrist have been discussed from a phylogenetic, ontogenetic, anatomic-descriptive, and clinical point of view (Thilenius 1895; Corner 1898; Zrubecky 1960; Lewis 1970; Blauth and Schneider-Sickert 1976; et al.), but so far no studies of these joints have been undertaken with a view to investigating the functional connection between morphology and specific strain.

This study aims to establish the relationship between the form and the normal or disturbed functioning of three important joints of the human hand: the proximal wrist joint, the saddle joint of the thumb, and the metacarpophalangeal joints, and to evaluate the findings biomechanically and clinically.

The study of the proximal wrist joint focuses on the discus articularis radioulnaris distalis. Its normal functioning and factors leading to lesions of the articular disk are studied. The transfer of load from the forearm to the hand is analyzed in connection with the study of disk injury as a result of classical fracture of the radius.

The articular surfaces and capsular ligaments of the saddle joint of the thumb are studied with a view to establishing the influence of primary mechanical effects on the development of the degenerative alterations frequently observed in this joint.

The metacarpophalangeal joints are examined to establish whether morphological findings in the supporting tissues of the individual joints permit conclusions to be drawn with respect to the strain placed on individual fingers.

2 The Proximal Wrist Joint

2.1 Introduction

The shape of the proximal wrist joint may be termed articulatio ellipsoidea, and it is this shape that is one of the major reasons why the human hand is so flexible. The joint is also referred to as the articulatio radiocarpea, which reflects the immediate contact between the distal end of the radius and part of the proximal carpal bones. However, the articular disk situated between the end of the ulna and the ossa lunatum and triquetrum is just as important when the functioning and description of the proximal wrist joint as a whole is to be considered. From an anatomic point of view, the discus articularis is both phylogenetically and ontogenetically interesting. In

1

clinical literature, it is considered important in connection with joint alterations of the wrist that impair joint function and may often be traced to traumatic causes.

The comparative anatomical studies carried out by Flower (1885), Thilenius (1895), Wood Jones (1944), Mörike (1964), Lewis (1965, 1970, 1972), Lewis et al. (1970), and Corrucini (1977) generally refer to the "withdrawal" of the ulna from the base of the hand that is necessary for pronation and supination. The loss of articulation between the ossa triquetrum and pisiforme and the styloid process of the ulna is assumed to "necessitate" filling the gap with the discus articularis. According to Leboucp (1886) and Corner (1898), this is the rudiment of an ulnar, pisiform finger. Thilenius (1895) believes it to be the os intermedium antebrachii, which Henckel (1931) and Olivier (1962) give reason to doubt. Parsons (1900), Mörike (1964), and Lewis (1965, 1970) argue that the disk can be traced to development of dorsal and palmar ligaments or capsulate parts of the distal radioulnar joint. The ligaments or capsule are believed to move into the gap like a meniscus. A similar view is held by Meyer (1873).

The discus articularis may be described as crescent shaped or triangular, with the tip of the triangle against the ulnar styloid process and the base distal to the incisura ulnaris radii. According to R. Fick (1904, 1911), the disk is thicker at the dorsal and palmar edges than in the center. Its primary function is to guide the distal radioulnar joint by gliding on the caput ulnae during pronation and supination of the hand (Fick R. 1911; Taylor and Parsons 1938).

There are various interpretations in the literature for the discontinuity of the disk that is sometimes observed in the form of a slit or a hole. Meyer (1873), Poirier and Charpy (1911), and Haage (1973) consider the link between the proximal wrist joint and the distal radioulnar joint that is caused by such discontinuity to be in some cases an innate anatomic variant, in others an acquired development. Martinek (1977) maintains that innate discontinuities of the disk can be distinguished from acquired ones by examination of the proximal wrist joint using contrast medium. Mikić (1978), however, believes that a cleft or perforation is always an acquired morphological feature characterizing tissue degeneration of the disk due to aging.

R. Fick (1911) and Von Lanz and Wachsmuth (1959) discount the possibility that mechanical factors, in the form of compression of the disk, can cause disk lesions, but Lang (1942), Arendt (1955), and Haage (1973) believe that the disk is subjected to pressure forces when the hand and forearm are under physiological load. Hofmann (1959) shows, by way of split line and polarization optics methods, that the collagen fibers of the disk are aligned in such a way that they can withstand both dominant traction forces and additional compression.

Documented injuries to the discus articularis which appear after spraining or bruising the proximal wrist joint or after a classical fracture of the radius appear to be the result of a nonrecurrent, severe traction and compression stress.

The analysis of load transfer between the forearm and the hand is critical to the question of whether and to what extent the disk is subjected to compressive stress. According to the generally accepted theory (Von Lanz and Wachsmuth 1959), the membrana interossea antebrachii relays stress between the two bones of the forearm. Compressive stress on the hand is held to be transferred primarily to the radius. The fibers of the interosseous membrane between radius and ulna become taut as a result of the movement of the radius towards the elbow. These taut fibers relay the stress to the ulna, which then transfers stress to the humerus via the elbow joint. The same mechanism is assumed in the case of a distal fracture of the radius caused by falling onto the outstretched arm; in this case, further stress comes to bear on the radius because it has to absorb the impact shock of the accelerated body weight due to the action of falling.

Pauwels (1963), however, disregards the transfer of load from the radius to the ulna via the membrana interossea in his calculation of stress distribution in the elbow joint. He justifies this by hypothesizing that the component of axial stress transferred via the membrane to the ulna is very low when the elbow joint is subjected to compressive stress. Morphological studies of the fetal and embryonic membrana interossea (Reinbach 1952) and the results of experimentally induced classical fracture of the radius (Frykman 1967, Nikolić et al. 1975) also fail to support the generally accepted theory of the function of the membrane. Halls and Travill (1964) and Rossak (1965, 1970) carried out compressive stress measurements of the elbow joint, and they conclude that the membrana interossea antebrachii does not function as a transferrer of load. However, these authors carried out their experiments under static conditions and shortcomings could also be observed in their methodology; their results, therefore, may not be evaluated without reservations.

In the first section of this study, macroscopic and microscopic investigation of the discus articularis of the fetus, the newborn child, and the adult, and split line examination of the joint surfaces of the os lunatum and the caput ulnae will be described and analyzed with respect to evidence of physiological compressive stress on the discus articularis.

Arthrographic and macroscopic examination of the disk is presented to establish the frequency of discontinuity of the disk and possible causes of such discontinuity.

Classical fracture of the radius is experimentally induced under dynamic conditions to establish the relevance of the membrana interossea for the transfer of kinetic energy.

Under the same experimental conditions, a clearer definition of the function of the membrane is attempted by establishing the kinetic energy transferred by radius and ulna when the membrane is intact and when it has been severed.

2.2 Material and Methods

The proximal wrist joints of 50 adults (aged 30 to 91), 6 children (aged about 3 to 4), and 10 newborns form the material basis.

2.2.1 Arthrographic and Macroscopic Examinations

In order to obtain a first X-ray picture of the closed joint of the articulatio radiocarpea and any communication with neighboring joints, a watery contrast medium (Urografin 65%) was injected into the joint. The adult hands came from the dissecting room and most of the soft tissue had been removed. The Urografin (1–3 ml) was introduced dorsally and radially into the intact joint capsule. The children's hands retained the soft tissue and the contrast medium was injected through the skin and soft tissue. To make sure the contrast medium was distributed throughout the joint capsule, the hands were passively moved without disturbing the joints. Dorsopalmar X-ray films were prepared. The roentgenograms were made with direct-exposure films (Kodak Definix Medical).

The radiocarpal joint was opened radially by severing the ligamentum collaterale radiale and gradually opening the capsule from the dorsal and palmar sides. This prevented any injury to the

3

discus articularis, situated against the ulna. The disk itself was prepared in situ. The ulnar collateral ligament was not severed. The proximal and distal joint surfaces were macroscopically examined and disk lesions and cartilage alterations photographed.

Where there was found to be a lesion of the discus articularis, the affected place was marked by inserting a short metal wire into the slit or perforation. The proximal and distal joint surfaces were then rejoined and another roentgenogram taken in dorsopalmar position. The distal radio-ulnar joint was opened and examined from the proximal side, without removing the discus articularis.

2.2.2 Production and Documentation of Split Lines

The course of the split lines was established on ten macroscopically intact distal articular surfaces (os scaphoideum, os lunatum, and os triquetrum), and ten intact ulnar heads. Ten further specimens were examined where there was degenerative cartilage damage to the os lunatum and the caput ulnae. The split lines were made according to the method described by Konermann (1971). The fixed material is soaked in water for several hours. The articular surface is covered with poster paint and pricked "blindly" with a sharp needle. The needle is always introduced into the cartilage at right angles to the articular surface. The paint is removed. The visible lines are photographed and the resulting picture is enlarged 4–5 times and copied onto transparent paper. The final drawing of the split line pattern shows the lines more widely spaced than in the original. Omission of some lines makes the general picture clearer and facilitates interpretation of the pattern.

2.2.3 Production and Histological Examination of Sawn Sections

Histological examination was carried out on disks from 15 adults, 4 children, and 8 newborns. The material had been fixed in an alcohol-formalin solution. The disks were embedded in Paraplast and cut lengthwise in the radioulnar orientation. Eleven further disks were histologically examined, together with the caput ulnae and the radial connection point. Where necessary, the sawn sections were decalcified in an EDTA solution for 4–6 weeks at 37 °C, and then embedded. Degenerative alteration of the cartilage of the os lunatum and the caput ulnae was examined in four cases each.

The sections cut from isolated articular disks were 7–9 μm thick; those from bone material were 10–15 μm thick. All material was stained with hematoxylin-eosin, azan, Goldner, and resorcin-fuchsin-van Gieson.

Frontal sections sawed through the distal end of the radius, the discus articularis, and the caput ulnae were prepared from five adult and two newborns joints. Material was deep-frozen and cut with a band saw to prevent the tissue from tearing.

2.2.4 Experiments

The Transfer of Kinetic Energy in the Forearm and the Experimental Induction of Forearm Fractures. Special apparatus was constructed to carry out measurements and to induce fractures of prepared forearms (Fig. 1)[1]. The forearms, which had previously been used in dissection courses, were prepared in the following way before being placed in the steel frame of the apparatus. Both forearm bones were sawn through, either 5 cm above the proximal wrist joint or 5 cm below the elbow joint. Where the bones had been sawn through, the marrow was scooped out of the hollow. The measuring probe or gauges consisted of two brass cylinders (2 cm high, 1.5 cm in diameter) that would not bend or twist, with a central metal rod with a slit in the middle (Fig. 2). The central metal rod in each cylinder contained four resistance strain gauges connected in

---

[1] Experiments were carried out with the cooperation of Dr. A. Brade and Dr. E. Hiss of the Kiel University Orthopedic Clinic.

My thanks are due to Prof. Dr. W. Blauth, Director of the Kiel University Orthopedic Clinic, for making it possible to carry out the experiments.

4

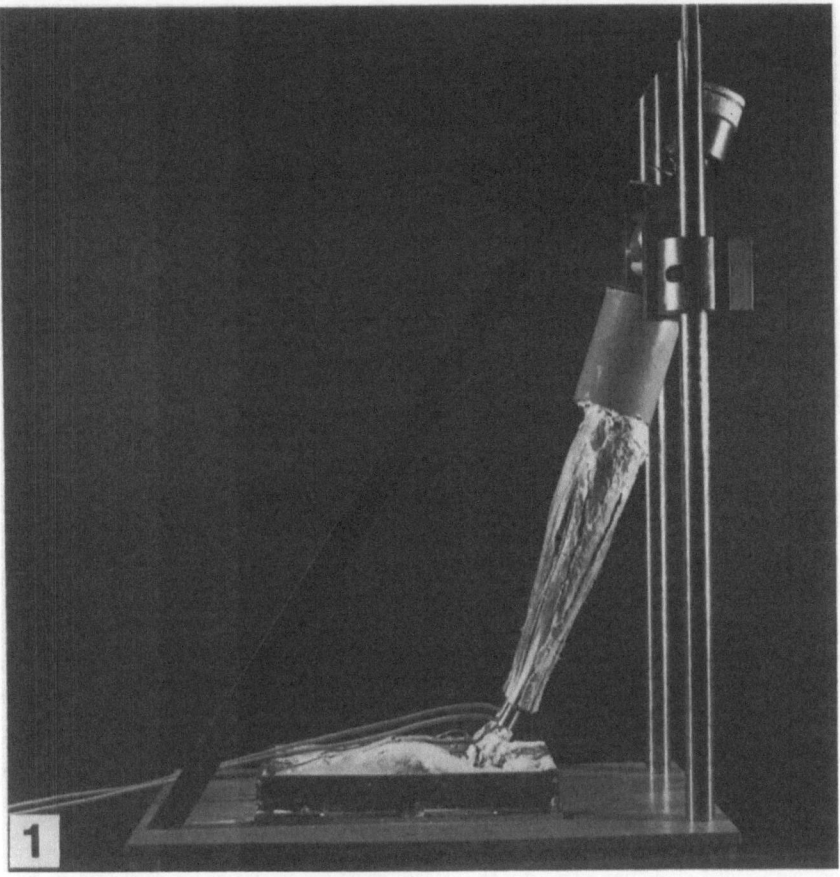

Fig. 1. Apparatus with arm secured. The stump of the humerus is plastered centrally into a plastic cylinder, the hand plastered in an aluminum tray. The two measuring gauges are glued into the forearm bones below the membrana interossea

a closed bridge circuit (Fig. 3). The calibrated brass gauges were implanted in the marrow cavity and fixed with bone glue.

All the muscles of the upper arm were removed and the humerus sawed off 10–15 cm proximal to the articulatio cubiti. The stump of the humerus was fixed in a rigid plastic cylinder (10 cm high, 6.5 cm in diameter) in plaster. In order to produce the axial transfer of energy necessary for the experiment, the humerus had to be centred in the plastic cylinder. This was achieved by introducing a screw into the cylinder from the end. The screw was advanced into the marrow cavity of the humerus and then removed when the plaster had set. The distal end of the hand was plastered into an aluminum tray as far as the metacarpal diaphyses. The elbow and the proximal wrist joints were freely movable. Prepared in this way, the arm was secured in the steel frame of the test apparatus. The aluminum tray was screwed down to the base plate. The base of the plastic cylinder was screwed into a bolt running at right angles to the vertical steel frame. The bolt had almost frictionless freedom of movement around the horizontal axis. The angle of extension of the proximal wrist joint could be increased or decreased by altering the position of the arm in the steel frame. This was achieved by temporarily loosening the aluminum tray and changing the height of the metal bolt holding the humerus.

Kinetic energy was brought to bear on the arm by hitting the cushioned end of the metal bolt with a hammer. The impulse was measured on a double beam oscillograph via carrier fre-

5

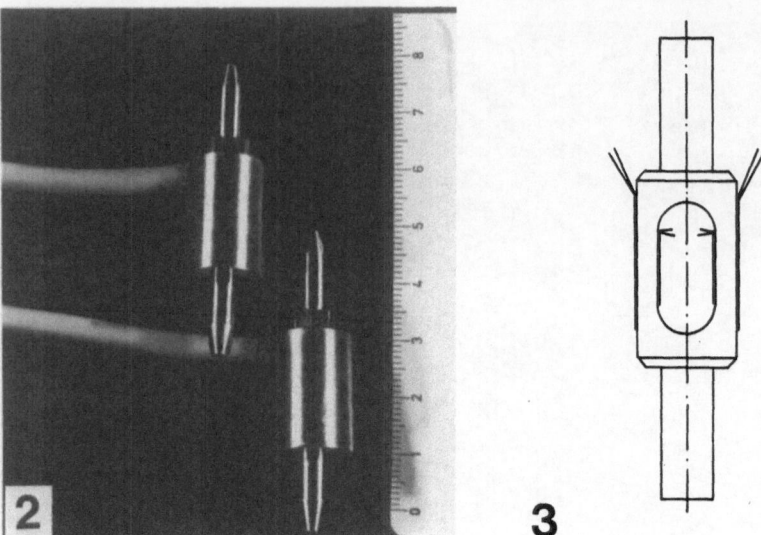

Fig. 2. Cylindrical measuring gauges that were implanted in the radius and ulna. The two metal tips were glued into the bone marrow cavity

Fig. 3. Cross-section of a measuring gauge without the brass sleeve. In the central slit of the stainless steel rod, there are 4 resistance strain gauges connected in a closed bridge circuit. Under load, the slit section of the rod is elastically deformed outwards

quency amplifiers. Measuring curves were photographed from the oscillograph screen with a miniature camera (black and white negative film, 15 DIN, aperture 5.6, exposure 1 sec).

Measurements were carried out on eight prepared arms. In six of them, the measuring gauges were implanted distally. The position of the wrist joint was varied between 60° and 80° dorsal extension, with radial abduction of 5° to 15°. Measurements were taken for each arm in zero position and with 15°, 30°, and 45° pronation, and 15°, 30°, 45°, and 60° supination. Thereafter, the membrana interossea antebrachii was completely severed and the measurements repeated. In the two other arms, the measuring gauges were implanted proximally and measurements taken with the membrane intact for 70° and 80° extension in the proximal wrist joint.

For evaluation of the measurements, prints were made from the negatives of the oscillograph curves. In order to calculate the proportional transfer of kinetic energy from the upper arm to the two forearm bones[2], the maximum amplitude of the two single-peaked curves was measured in cm. Values obtained were expressed as percentages, where the sum of the two amplitudes was taken to be 100%. A linear regression analysis with a second degree polynomial was carried out for the data arising from distally implanted measuring gauges ($n = 6$).

Fourteen arms were used in experiments to induce distal fracture of the radius. Prior to the experiments, lateral and dorsopalmar roentgenograms and arthrograms of the proximal wrist joints of these arms were prepared. The arms were then introduced into the apparatus as described above, except that no measuring gauges were implanted. In the case of two of the arms, the membrana interossea antebrachii was severed after the arm had been secured in the apparatus, but the capsule and ligaments of the proximal and distal radioulnar joint were left intact. In all cases, the arms were placed in a 45° pronation position. The proximal wrist joint was extended 60°−80° dorsally. The kinetic energy required to induce a fracture was provided by a pendulum hitting the impact surface (pendulum kilogram-force 5 kp = 49.05 N). The parameters of pendulum weight and height

---

[2] This evaluation method is based on the assumption that the energy/time course of radius and ulna are approximately the same (publication in preparation).

of fall allowed the energy applied to be calculated for each experiment. Values lay between 2940 and 5880 joule. After each experiment, another lateral and dorsopalmar roentgenogram and an arthrogram were prepared for the proximal wrist joint. The articulatio radiocarpea was then opened and examined macroscopically. The articulatio cubiti was also dissected and examined.

2.3 Results

2.3.1 Arthrographic, Macroscopic, and Split Line Findings

The arthrographic analysis showed that in 16 of the 50 proximal wrist joints examined, only the radiocarpal joint capsule was filled with contrast medium. Dorsopalmar arthrograms show the joint cavity as a crescent-shaped line of contrast medium, proximally convex. In nine of the 16 cases, a kind of pocket in the joint cavity could be observed in the region of the ulnar styloid process. This pocked varied in shape and size. Two other hands showed contrast medium not only in the cavity of the articulatio radiocarpea, but also in the articulatio ossis pisiformis. The 32 remaining hands showed accessory filling of the articulatio radioulnaris distalis cavity, and in 12 of these the contrast medium was again found in the pisiform joint cavity. Contrast medium in the distal radioulnar joint and in the radiocarpal and intercarpal joints was found in seven of the 32 hands. In five of these seven, the crevice between the os lunatum and the os scaphoideum contained contrast medium, in the other two, the medium was found between the os lunatum and os triquetrum. An ulnar recess in the proximal wrist joint cavity was found in 17 of the 32 cases.

The arthrograms of the children's hands were all much the same. In each case, contrast medium was found only in the cavity of the articulatio radiocarpea.

Of the 50 proximal wrist joints opened and examined, 28 showed no macroscopically visible degenerative alteration of the articular surface. The surface of the discus articularis was smooth on the carpal side, while the surface on the ulnar side was often found to be rough. Eleven disks had a zone that appeared thin to the naked eye. Twenty-nine of the wrist joints examined were found to have a dorsopalmar fissure (Fig. 4) or an almost circular hole (Fig. 5) in the radial part of the discus articularis. In 12 joints where the discus articularis had a large hole, the articular surfaces showed varying degrees of cartilage damage. On the distal side of the joint, this damage occurred in the form of clearly defined dorsoulnar spot lesions (Fig. 6a), or as larger cartilage defects covering the whole ulnar surface of the os lunatum (Fig. 6b). On the proximal side of the joint, the articular surface of the caput ulnae had degenerated in the palmarradial zone (Fig. 7a, b). In three cases, it could be seen that the radial part of the ulna protruded through the perforated discus articularis. In these cases, the distal radioulnar joint also showed signs of degeneration (Fig. 8a).

The split lines in the articular cartilage of an intact os lunatum are characterized by a radioulnar set of the lines in the palmarradial area (Fig. 8b). A second cluster of lines describes a curve around a dorsoulnar attractive singular point. A repulsive singular point lies at the ulnar tip of the lunate articular surface[3].

---

[3] The term attractive singular point is used to designate a point in the pattern around which the split lines cluster like hairpins. A repulsive singular point is characterized by the split lines' divergence from this point (Pauwels 1959).

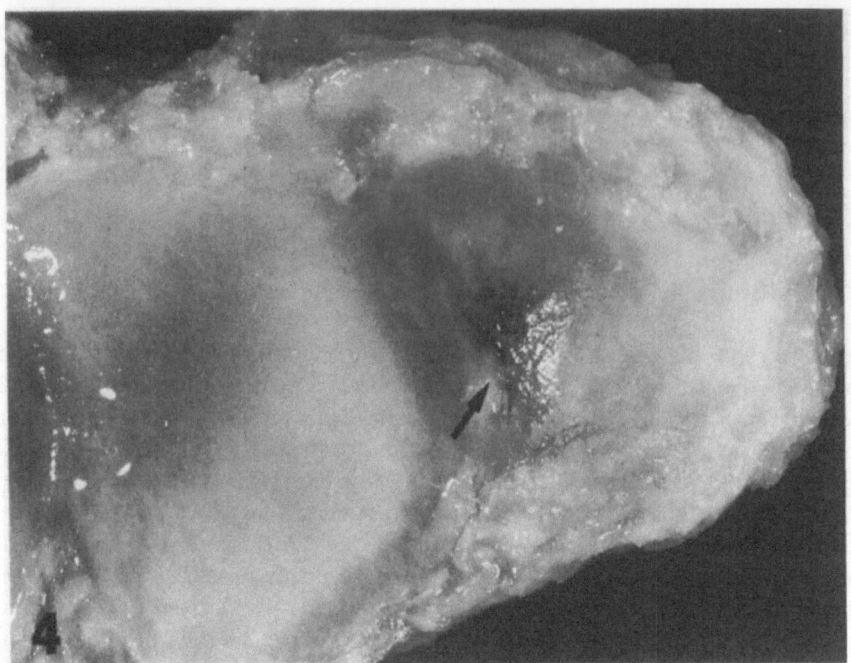

Fig. 4. View from above of the carpal surface of the left discus articularis of a 63-year-old woman. Dorsopalmar disk fissure (*arrow*) at the point of radial connection (radius on the *left* in the photograph)

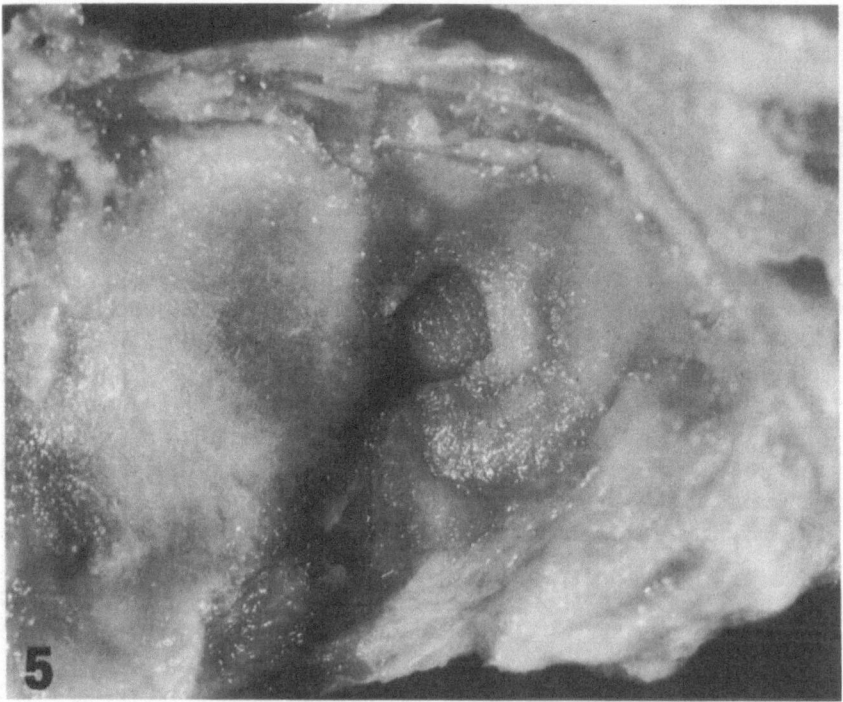

Fig. 5. View from above of the carpal surface of the left discus articularis of a 77-year-old woman. Perforation of the disk at the point of radial insertion. Caput ulnae visible through the perforation

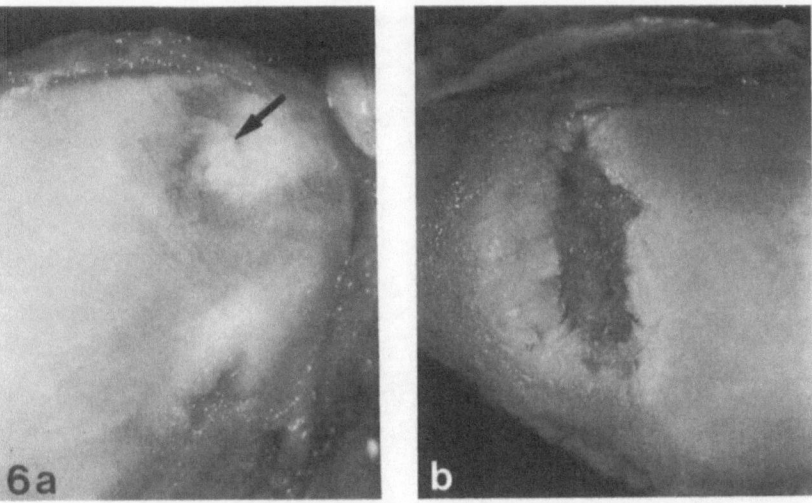

Fig. 6. Cartilage deficiencies on the os lunatum. *a* Right os lunatum of an 81-year-old woman. Minor lesion of the cartilage in the dorsoulnar zone (*arrow*). *b* View of the left os lunatum of a 59-year-old man. Large area of cartilage destruction in the ulnar part

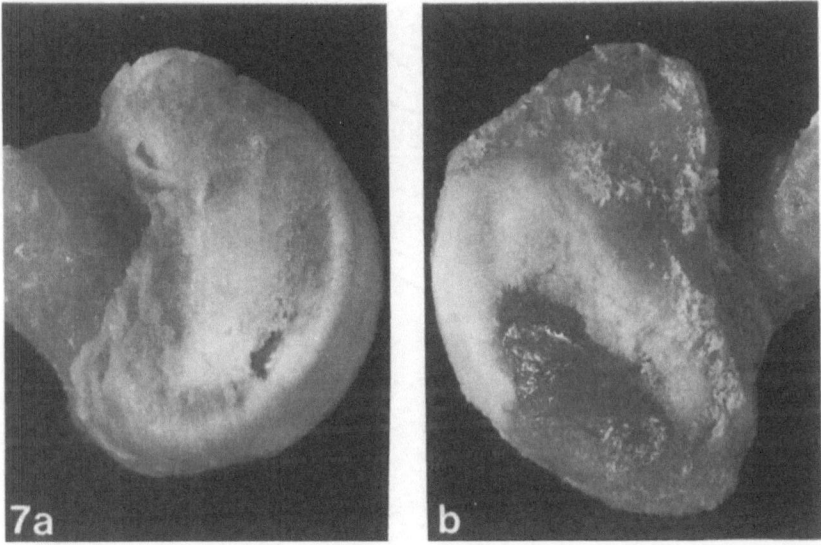

Fig. 7. Cartilage deficiencies on the caput ulnae. *a* Top distal view of the right caput ulnae of a 70-year-old woman. Localized palmarradial cartilage lesion. *b* Distal view of the left caput ulnae of a 78-year-old woman with a large area of cartilage destruction

The split lines of the 10 ossa lunata examined that gave evidence of cartilage degeneration showed the same course of lines, at least in those cases where the damage was in the form of a small spot lesion. The cartilage deficiency was situated close to the dorsoulnar attractive singular point.

9

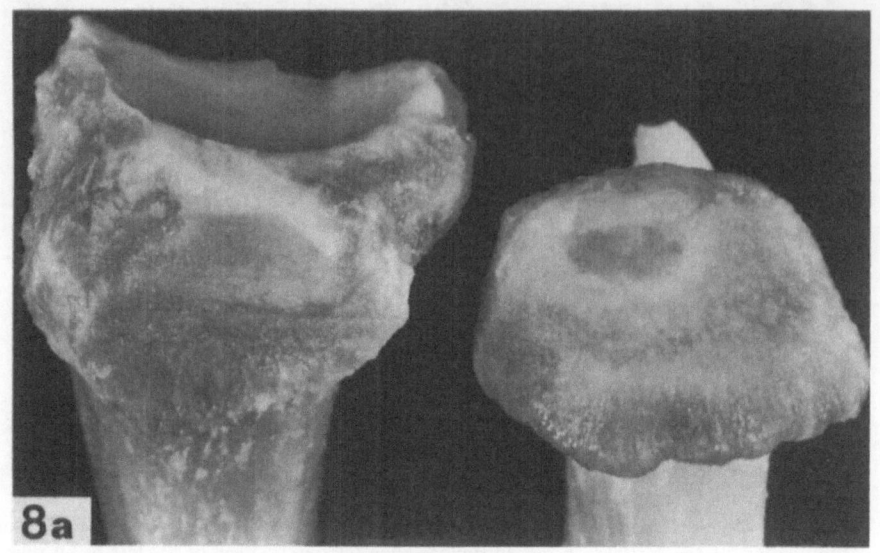

DORSAL

ULNAR

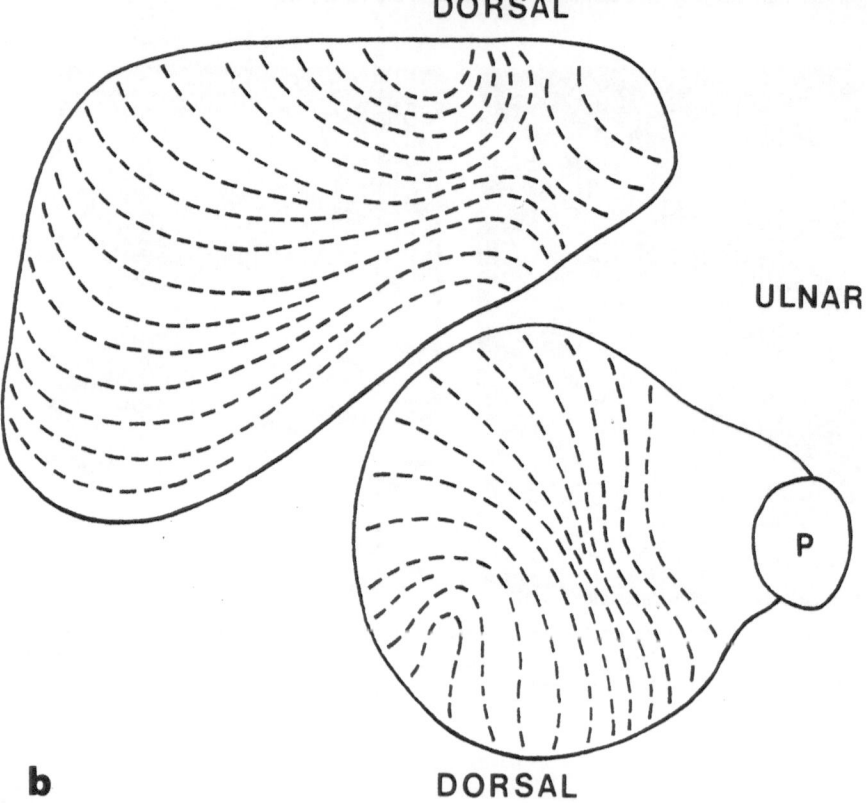

P

b　　　　　　　　**DORSAL**

Fig. 8. *a* Right distal radioulnar joint of a 67-year-old man. The articular surfaces of the radius (*left*) and the ulna (*right*) show arthritic degeneration. Ulnar head with osteophytic proliferations. *b* Split lines on the os lunatum (*top*) and the caput ulnae (*below; P*, styloid process). On the os lunatum there is an attractive singular point in the dorsoulnar region, on the caput ulnae in the palmarradial zone

The split lines of the caput ulnae run in a dorsopalmar direction. They form an attractive singular point in the palmarradial zone of the articular surface (Fig. 8b). Analysis of the split line pattern of the caput ulnae where cartilage deficiencies occurred was found to be very difficult. Even where only very small macroscopic lesions could be seen in the palmarradial zone, there were only a few dorsopalmar split lines in the ulnar part of the cartilage that could be seen, running parallel to each other.

2.3.2 Histological Findings

The central part of the discus articularis of newborns has closely packed bundles of collagen fibers running in a radioulnar direction. Such a clear directional pattern of the fibers is not visible at the ulnar and radial edges of the disk. The fibroblasts under the smooth carpal and ulnar surfaces of the disk are oblong; those in the central area are round. The disk itself is almost equally thick everywhere, except for the reinforced dorsal and palmar edges.

In the four disks from the hands of children examined in this study, the central collagen fibers were found to lie in a radioulnar direction. Between the bundles of collagen fibers there were fibrocytes and also cartilage cells, singly or lying in small clusters. The carpal and ulnar disk surfaces were smooth and the disk appeared to be uniformly thick.

Of the 15 histolocically examined disks from adult hands, 12 were clearly thinner in the radial zone than elsewhere; this could be seen from radioulnar sections. It is in this zone that fissures or perforations of the discus articularis occur. Three of the disks examined had a fissure in the disk. The radial zone, where the lesion was situated, was not noticeably thinner than the rest of the disk in these cases, however (Fig. 9). In all the disks examined, the collagen fiber bundles ran in a radioulnar direction. The central radial zone of the disks showed only chondrocytes (Fig. 10).

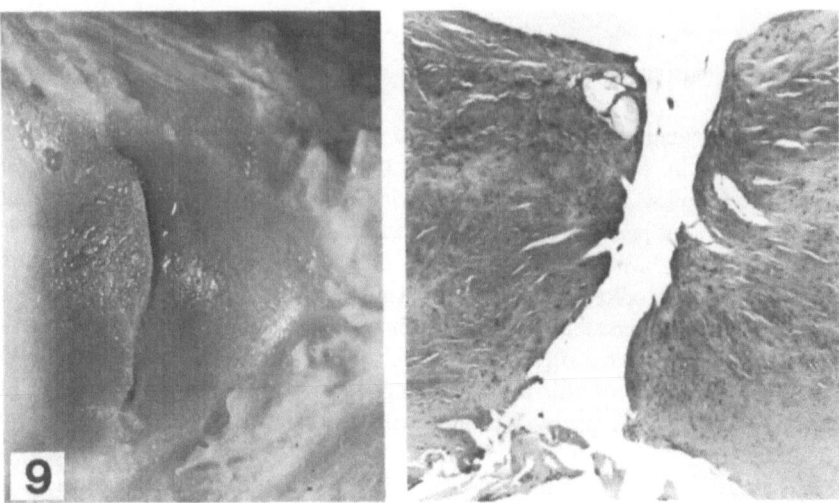

Fig. 9. Top view of the carpal surface of the left discus articularis of a 59-year-old woman (*left*). The disk has a fissure radially. A histological section (*right*) in a radioulnar direction shows that the disk is thick close to the fissure. Hematoxylin-eosin, 10 µm; × 25

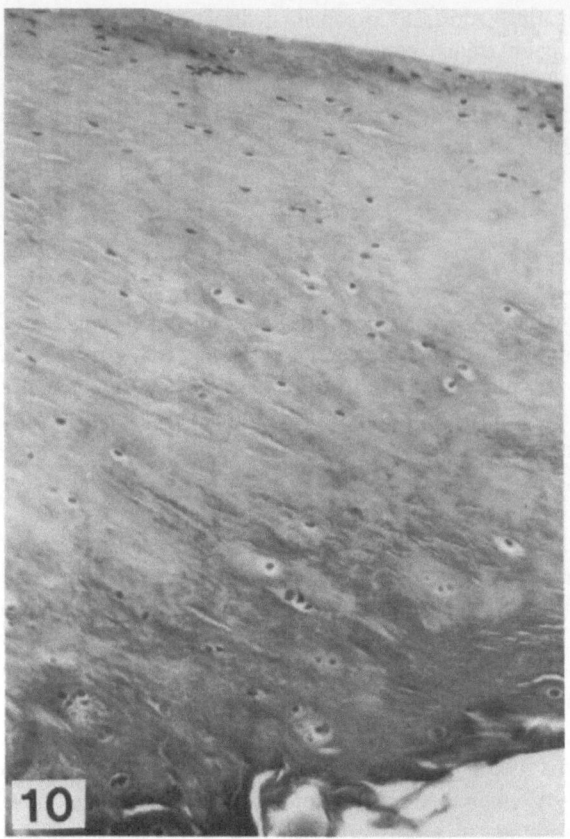

Fig. 10. Central radial section from the disk of a 77-year-old woman. Numerous cartilage cells between the collagen fibers. The carpal surface (*top*) is smooth, the ulnar surface (*bottom*) rough. Azan, 8 μm; × 70

The carpal disk surface was smooth in all cases, and the ulnar surface rough and uneven.

The discus articularis is fastened in two places at the distal end of the ulna: collagen fibers run to the tip and to the radial side of the styloid process, and the disk is anchored to a hollow at the base of the styloid process by a strong band of fibers. Between the points of insertion there is vascularized, loose-knit connective tissue.

The articular surface of the caput ulnae on the side where it meets the discus articularis was found to consist of hyaline cartilage in newborns and young children. In adults this surface consisted of either hyaline cartilage alone, or of a base layer of hyaline cartilage which gradually gave way to a superimposed layer of more fibrous cartilage. The thickness of this upper cartilage layer varied considerably (Fig. 11). In a few cases the caput ulnae was covered with a purely fibrous cartilage layer with very few cells.

Degenerative alteration of the articular surfaces of the os lunatum and the caput ulnae were found to be reflected in complete loss of the cartilage layer in some places and in scaliness or fibrillation of the remaining cartilage. The cartilage surface was uneven and broken, and cartilage cell clusters lay close to the surface (Fig. 12).

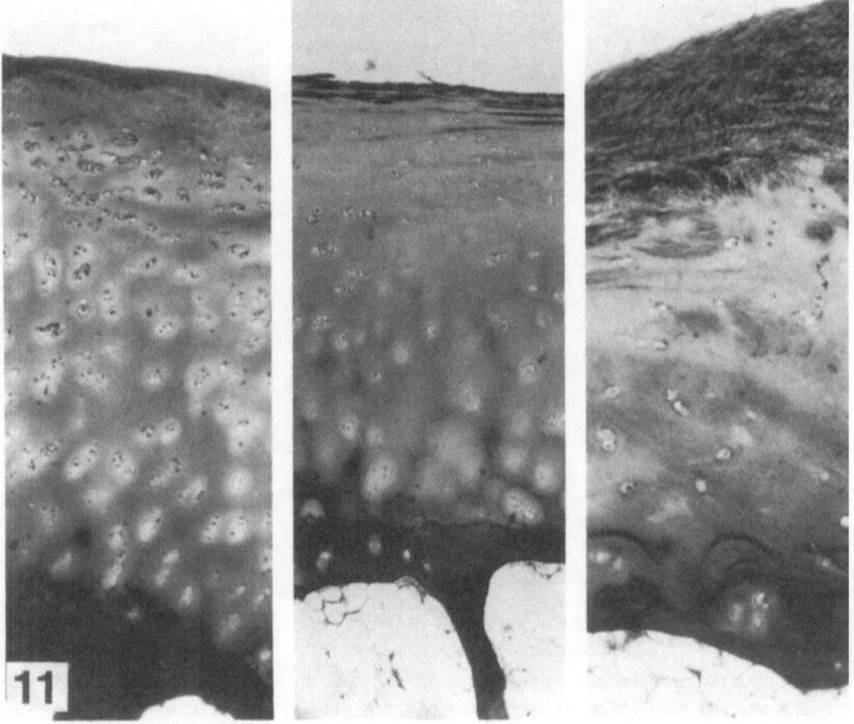

Fig. 11. Cartilage on the caput ulnae of three adults. *Left,* a layer consisting only of hyaline cartilage; center, hyaline cartilage with a thin top layer of fibers; *right*, hyaline cartilage and fibrous layer equally thick, Goldner, 8 μm; × 65

2.3.3 Experimental Results

The Transfer of Kinetic Energy from the Upper Arm to the Hand. The relative kinetic energy transferred from the upper arm to the two long bones of the forearm, as measured by distally and proximally implanted measuring gauges, is given in percentages in Table 1. The percentages calculated for the radius are based on linear regression analysis with a second degree polynomial.

Where the membrana interossea antebrachii was intact, the percentage of kinetic energy transmitted through the radius increased from 81% to 83.8% for positions from 0° to 45° pronation (Fig. 13). In supination of the forearm, the amount of energy transferred by the radius dropped steadily to 57.6% at 60° supination.

When the membrana interossea antebrachii had been severed, the radius transmitted 84.8% of the total kinetic energy in zero position (Fig. 14). This percentage rose to 86.8% at 45° pronation. The value for the radius dropped to 61% at 60° supination.

Measurement of kinetic energy via proximally implanted measuring gauges in two arms (arms 7 and 8) showed values of about 80% for the radius during pronation. The percentage of kinetic energy transmitted through the radius was here also found to drop with increasing supination, until the value for the ulna rose to 40% (arm 7) and 34% (arm 8).

13

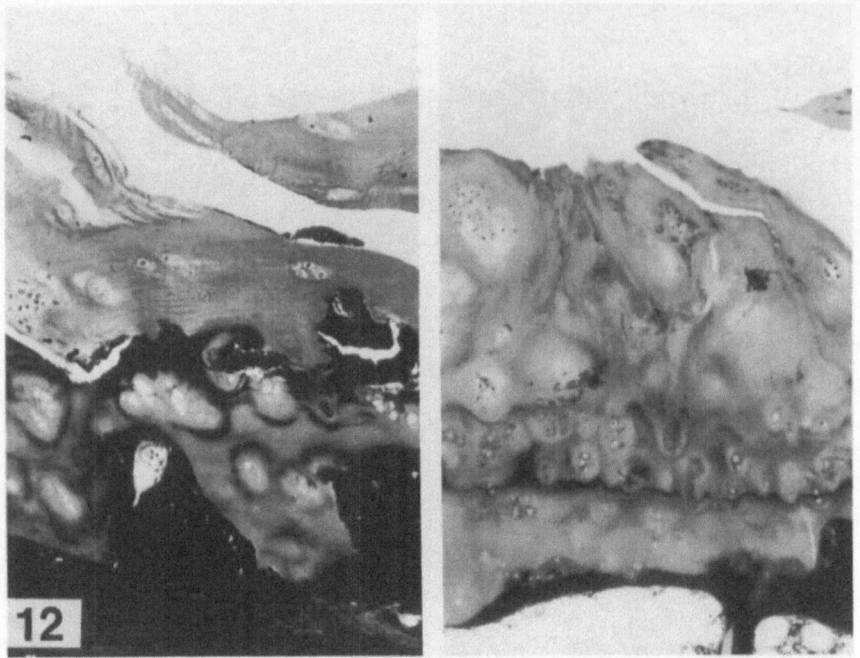

Fig. 12. Cartilage degeneration of the os lunatum (*left*) and the caput ulnae (*right*) of a 72-year-old man. The articular cartilage is broken up and chondrocyte clusters can be seen near the surface of the caput ulnae. Goldner, 8 μm; × 80

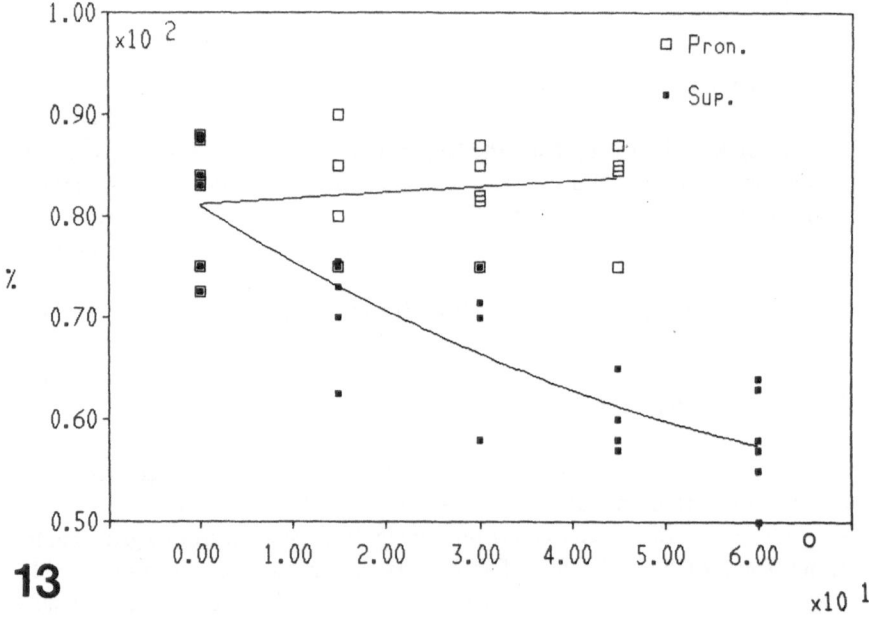

Fig. 13. Graph showing percentage of kinetic energy transmitted by the radius with membrane intact. Linear regression analysis based on measurements with six arms

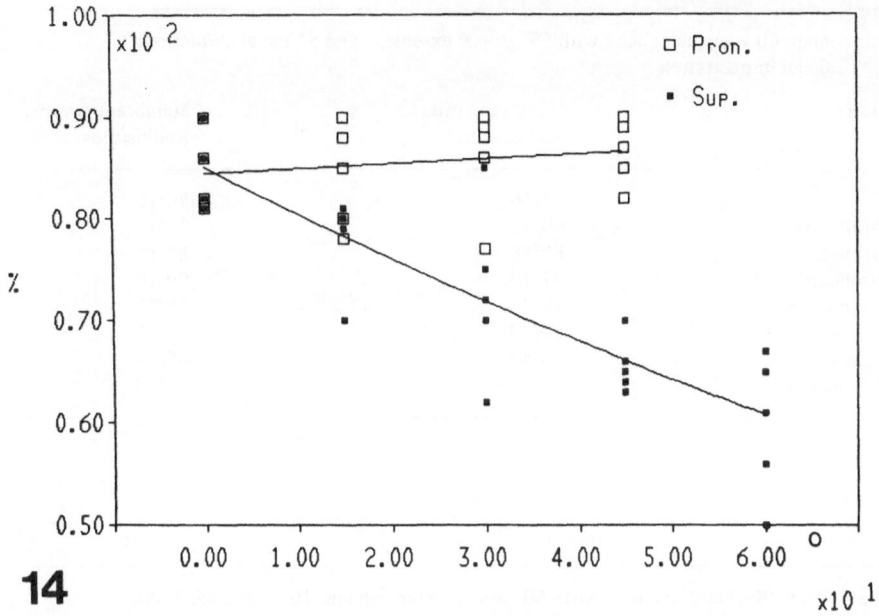

Fig. 14. Graph showing percentage of kinetic energy transmitted by the radius with severed membrana interossea. Linear regression analysis based on measurements with six arms

Forearm Fractures. A distal fracture of the radius was observed in nine of the 14 arms used in experiments to induce fractures (see Table 2). In seven of the nine cases, fractures were intraarticular, affecting the radiocarpal and/or the distal radioulnar joint. In four cases, this was combined with severance of the ulnar styloid process. One arm was found to be broken at the distal end of the radius and at the os scaphoideum. The two arms in which the membrana interossea antebrachii had been severed (arms 13 and 14) were found to have suffered a loco typico radius fracture. In one case (arm 12), not only the distal end of the radius but also the ulna was broken close to the proximal wrist joint.

Table 1. Transmitted kinetic energy (%) with intact and severed membrana interossea antebrachii

Arm 1: Woman, 79 years, left; hand with 70° dorsal extension and 5° radial abduction; distal implantation

Position	Membrane intact Radius/ulna	Membrane severed Radius/ulna
0°	83/17	86/14
15° pronation	80/20	80/20
30° pronation	87/13	90/10
45° pronation	87/13	89/11
15° supination	75/25	70/30
30° supination	70/30	85/15
45° supination	60/40	70/30
60° supination	50/50	50/50

15

Arm 2: Man, 60 years, left; hand with 69° dorsal extension and 5° radial abduction; distal implantation

Position	Membrane intact Radius/ulna	Membrane severed Radius/ulna
0°	84/16	90/10
15° pronation	90/10	90/10
30° pronation	82/18	89/11
45° pronation	87/13	90/10
15° supination	70/30	79/21
30° supination	70/30	75/25
45° supination	60/40	66/34
60° supination	57/43	61/39

Arm 3: Man, 90 years, left; hand with 60° dorsal extension and 10° radial abduction; distal implantation

Position	Membrane intact Radius/ulna	Membrane severed Radius/ulna
0°	87.5/12.5	86/14
15° pronation	80/20	85/15
30° pronation	85/15	88/12
45° pronation	85/15	85/15
15° supination	70/30	80/20
30° supination	71.5/28.5	72/28
45° supination	60/40	63/37
60° supination	55/45	56/44

Arm 4: Man, 90 years, right; hand with 75° dorsal extension and 5° radial abduction; distal implantation

Position	Membrane intact Radius/ulna	Membrane severed Radius/ulna
0°	88/12	90/10
15° pronation	85/15	88/12
30° pronation	85/15	86/14
45° pronation	87/13	90/10
15° supination	73/27	81/19
30° supination	70/30	75/25
45° supination	65/35	70/30
60° supination	58/42	67/33

Arm 5:   Woman, 72 years, left; hand with 80° dorsal extension and 10° radial abduction; distal implantation

Position	Membrane intact Radius/ulna	Membrane severed Radius/ulna
0°	75/25	81/19
15° pronation	75/25	78/22
30° pronation	75/25	77/23
45° pronation	75/25	82/18
15° supination	62.5/37.5	70/30
30° supination	58/42	62/38
45° supination	58/42	65/35
60° supination	64/36	65/35

Arm 6:   Man, 58 years, right; hand with 80° dorsal extension and 10° radial abduction; distal implantation

Position	Membrane intact Radius/ulna	Membrane severed Radius/ulna
0°	72.5/27.5	82/18
15° pronation	80/20	78/22
30° pronation	81.5/18.5	88/12
45° pronation	84.5/15.5	87/13
15° supination	75.5/24.5	79/21
30° supination	75/25	70/30
45° supination	57/43	64/36
60° supination	63/37	65/35

Arm 7:   Man, 66 years, left; hand with 80° dorsal extension and 5° radial abduction; proximal implantation

Position	Membrane intact Radius/ulna
0°	73/27
15° pronation	78/22
30° pronation	83/17
45° pronation	82/18
15° supination	71/29
30° supination	66.5/33.5
45° supination	64/36
60° supination	60/40

Arm 8: Man, 69 years, right; hand with 75° dorsal extension and 10° radial abduction; proximal implantation

Position	Membrane intact Radius/ulna
0°	79/21
15° pronation	80.5/19.5
30° pronation	86/14
45° pronation	82/18
15° supination	75.5/24.5
30° supination	72/28
45° supination	66/34
60° supination	66/34

Table 2. Experimentally induced fractures of 14 arms

Arm			Result
1:	Man, 79 years;	left	Distal fracture of the radius including radiocarpal joint, severance of the ulnar styloid process
2:	Man, 70 years;	right	Distal fracture of the radius including radiocarpal joint, severance of the ulnar styloid process
3:	Man, 70 years;	right	Distal fracture of the radius, fracture of the os scaphoideum
4:	Woman, 65 years;	left	Distal fracture of the radius including radiocarpal joint and distal radioulnar joint, severance of the ulnar styloid process
5:	Woman, 82 years;	left	Distal fracture of the radius
6:	Man, 73 years;	right	Fracture of the caput radii, distal dislocation of the ulna
7:	Woman, 75 years;	left	Distal fracture of the radius including radiocarpal joint and distal radioulnar joint, severance of the ulnar styloid process
8:	Sex and age unknown;	right	Fracture of the caput radii
9:	Woman, 91 years;	right	Fracture of radius and ulna, fracture of the os scaphoideum
10:	Woman, 86 years;	left	Fracture of the os scaphoideum, fracture of olecranon
11:	Man, 55 years;	left	Fracture of the os scaphoideum, os triquetrum, and os capitatum
12:	Woman, 78 years;	left	Distal fracture of the radius including radiocarpal joint and distal radioulnar joint, distal fracture of the ulna
13:	Woman, 78 years;	left	Distal fracture of the radius including radiocarpal joint
14:	Woman, 86 years;	right	Distal fracture of the radius including radiocarpal joint and distal radioulnar joint

2.4 Discussion

The Evidence of Arthrography in Evaluating the Importance of the Discus Articularis.
Referring to the proximal wrist joint as the point of articulation between the distal
end of the radius and the proximal root of the hand is an incomplete way of describing the anatomic relations between the bones of the forearm and the hand. The importance of the "ulnar half" of the joint is often only noticed, as pointed out by
Lang (1942), when recent or old traumatic damage to the joint leads to considerable
loss of function.

The discus articularis plays a central role in the "ulnar compartment of the proximal wrist joint" (H. Haage 1979, personal communication). The disk fills the gap that
appears to lie between the caput ulnae and the proximal bones of the wrist, as is
apparent on a roentgenogram. Haage (1966, 1973) and Haage and Cornelius (1966)
point out the particular advantages of contrast studies of the proximal wrist joint in
diagnosing the functioning of the discus articularis. Early arthrographic studies of the
proximal wrist joint were carried out by Rosenthal (1949), Kessler and Silberman
(1961), Thoms (1962), and Rösli (1963).

Arthrographic techniques permit not only the joint cavity of the articulatio
radiocarpea itself to be clearly shown, but also any connections between this cavity
and neighboring ones. Earlier descriptions of connections between the proximal wrist
joint cavity and that of the pisiform joint and/or the intercarpal joint recess (Haage
1966, 1973) were supported by the evidence of this study. The pocket sometimes
observed in various stages of development in the wrist cavity close to the ulnar styloid
process corresponds to the recessus ulnaris referred to in clinical literature. This is
usually described as a pocket on the volar side of the processus styloideus. The present
study gives no evidence to support the existence of a cartilagenous "meniscus ulno-
carpalis," as described by Lewis et al. (1970), Taleisnik (1976), and Poigenfürst and
Tuchmann (1978), which these authors maintain serves to separate the recessus ulnaris
from the wrist joint cavity.

According to Haage (1973), there are two possible explanations for the fact that
contrast medium reaches the articulatio radioulnaris distalis from the proximal wrist
joint cavity. The contrast medium usually passes into the radioulnar joint cavity via a
lesion in the discus articularis; however, there are alleged cases where the two joint
cavities are connected in spite of the disk being intact. Kessler and Silberman (1961)
also support this view, although they are not able to say how the contrast medium
passes from the wrist joint cavity to that of the neighboring joint. Anatomic dissection indicated that the two cavities can only connect by way of a discontinuity in the
discus articularis (Meyer 1873; Fick R. 1904; Poirier and Charpy 1911; Von Lanz and
Wachsmuth 1959). The results of the present study, founded on material provided by
the dissection room, support this hypothesis. In all cases examined where the contrast
medium was found to be present in the distal radioulnar joint, the medium had reached the cavity through the articular disk. Frequently this process was clearly indicated
in the arthrogram by a thin line of contrast medium connecting the two joint cavities;
this was confirmed by roentgenography (Fig. 15). In some cases, the radioulnar joint
cavity was full of contrast medium, but the arthrogram did not show a connection between the two cavities through the discus articularis (Fig. 16). In three such cases, the
discus articularis was almost uniformly thick, but macroscopic examination and cross-
checking by roentgenography indicated that a discontinuity of the disk was also

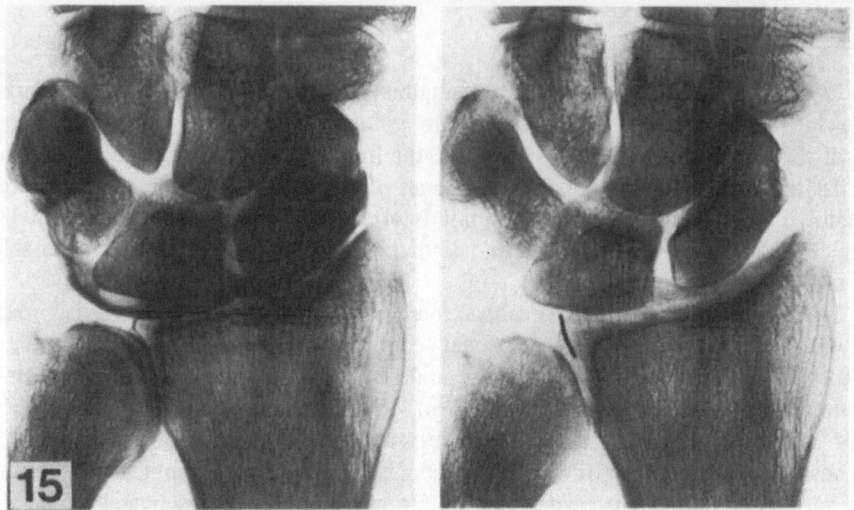

Fig. 15. Arthrogram (*left*) and control film (*right*) of the left proximal wrist joint of a 79-year-old woman, PA. The passage of contrast medium into the distal radioulnar joint is indicated by a thin line. The wire on the control film is in the disk fissure

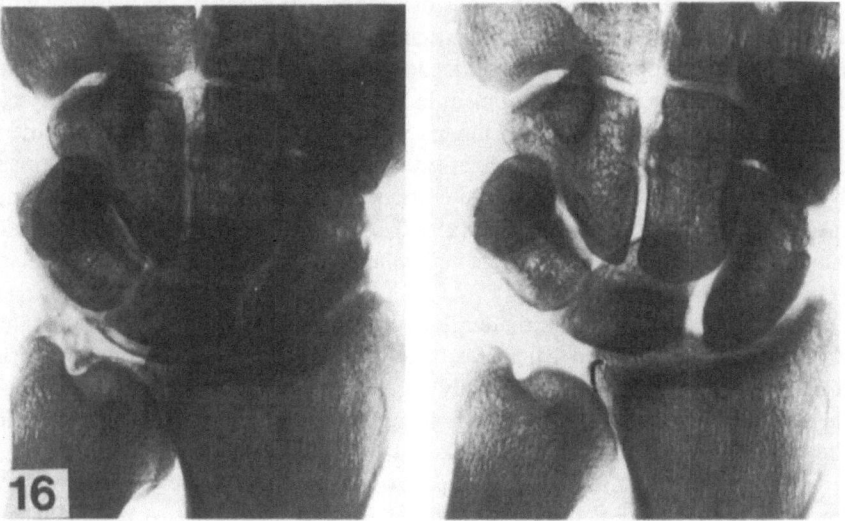

Fig. 16. Arthrogram (*left*) and control film (*right*) of the left proximal wrist joint of a 66-year-old man, PA. The distal radioulnar joint is filled with contrast medium. The connection between the joints is not visible in the arthrogram. The wire in the control film shows the position of the disk fissure through which the contrast medium reached the radioulnar joint

present. A short, narrow fissure was found to run in a dorsopalmar direction in the radial part of the disk. The edges of the fissure lay close together like lips. This seems to confirm the assumption of R. Fick (1904) that the contrast medium is introduced under pressure from the proximal wrist joint cavity into the cavity of the distal radio-ulnar joint. The rise in pressure in the wrist joint cavity causes the edges of the fissure in the disk to separate. They subsequently close tightly again. This kind of valve mechanism in a disk that appears intact on an arthrogram would explain the view held by Kessler and Silberman (1961) and Haage (1973), who believe that connection of the two cavities can occur for reasons other than a lesion in the discus articularis.

Frequency and Genesis of Discontinuity of the Discus Articularis. Various views are expounded in the literature with respect to the frequency, genesis, and evaluation of discontinuities of the discus articularis. The frequency of occurrence of disk perforation is given by Poirier and Charpy (1911) as 40.3%, by Von Lanz and Wachsmuth (1959) as 26%, by Haage (1973) as 33%, and by Weissman and Legsdinsch (1979) as 43%.

Examination of wrist joints from the dissection room carried out by Lewis et al. (1970) showed perforation of the discus articularis in over half the joints. In the course of the present study of 50 joints, the existence of a fissure or perforation was established in over 60% of cases ($n = 32$). These results, established for a population with a relatively high average age, imply that frequency of disk perforation increases with increasing age. First confirmation of this hypothesis is offered by the study carried out by Mikić (1978). He was able to show that no perforation is found up to the age of 20, that occasional cases arise in the next ten years, and that in later years a steady rise in cases of disk perforation may be observed. He interprets the perforation as an advanced stage of the natural degeneration of the disk tissue, which begins between the ages of 20 and 30. He discounts the possibility of innate discontinuity of the discus articularis. This view is not shared by Meyer (1873), Poirier and Charpy (1911), and Haage (1973), who consider a fissure in the disk to be a possible innate anatomic variant. Meyer (1873) sees the occasionally observed discontinuity of the disk as morphological evidence for his hypothesis that the disk developed from two separate menisci that gradually moved into the joint cavity. In the same way, Mörike (1964) maintains, on the basis of comparative anatomical investigations, that the discus articularis of the human wrist joint developed from a palmar and a dorsal ligament. These ligaments are found in numerous quadrupeds, where they function as guiding and restricting ligaments connecting the distal ends of the radius and ulna. Comparative anatomic and embryological studies by Lewis (1965, 1970), Lewis et al. (1970), and Kauer (1975) indicate that these hypotheses are not tenable. According to Lewis (1965, 1970), the articular disk developed from capsular parts of the distal radioulnar joint, that is, from a meniscus intraarticularis near the ulna which is regularly found in primates, and from the os daubentonii, which is still found in *Hylobates* as an individual bone lying between the caput ulnae and the os triquetrum. According to Kauer (1975), the discus articularis is part of a connective tissue system extending from the ulnar edge of the radius to the base of the os metacarpale V and continuing into the tendon sheath of the m. extensor carpi ulnaris. In the fetal specimens examined by Kauer (1975), which had a maximal crown-rump length of 230 mm, the discus articularis was a fibrous disk of uniform thickness lying between the caput ulnae and the ossa lunatum and triquetrum.

Similar results were obtained from the examination of newborns in the present study. The articular disk was found to be of uniform thickness, and fissure or perforation of the disk was not observed.

These findings imply that discontinuity of the disk is not an innate, but invariably an acquired, morphological feature. It therefore follows that Martinek's hypothesis

(1977) cannot be confirmed; he maintained that it was possible to distinguish arthrographically between innate and acquired disk deficiencies.

Causes of Disk Perforation: Compressive Strain on the Disk. As yet no answer has been presented to the question of what causes fissures or perforations in the disk. It has been postulated that malnutrition of the disk from changes in blood vessels (Lang 1942) or synovia (Arendt 1955) increases with age and may promote degeneration. Mechanical factors are also considered to lead to disk perforation. Mikić (1978) sees the rotatory movement in pronation and supination as a particular mechanical strain on the articular disk. He suggests that the double anchorage to the radius and the ulnar styloid process means that the disk is subjected to a "drilling effect" by the end of the ulna when the hand is turned.

Meyer (1873), R. Fick (1911), and Von Lanz and Wachsmuth (1959) do not believe that the disk is normally subjected to compressive stress that could lead to the development of a fissure or perforation of the disk. These authors hold the view that load on the hand is primarily transmitted only to the distal part of the radius. The stress is then taken up by the fibers of the membrana interossea antebrachii, which connect downward to the central part of the crista interossea of the radius, and these transfer the stress to the ulna. This is how pressure is then transferred via the ulna to the trochlea humeri which, according to R. Fick (1911), is better able to take the stress than the capitulum humeri. This type of load distribution in the forearm demonstrates the functional importance of the membrana interossea antebrachii, as set out and explained in anatomic textbooks, and also explains the downward direction of the membrane fibers. Similarly, the frequently occurring distal fracture of the radius in connection with falling onto the dorsally outstretched hand is due, according to Von Lanz and Wachsmuth (1959), to the transfer of load from the ulna to the radius via the membrana interossea.

In contradiction to these views, there are also observations and evidence in the literature to support the theory that the discus articularis is indeed subjected to compressive stress during physiological load on the hand and the forearm, and that stress leading to fracture of the radius also causes specific mechanical stress on the ulnar part of the proximal wrist joint.

Shepherd (1891) investigated anatomic dissection material and observed disk perforation and cartilage deficiencies of the os lunatum and the caput ulnae; he interpreted his findings as degenerative or traumatically induced alterations. Lang (1942) suggested that not only the rotatory traction stress that R. Fick (1904, 1911) considered of primary importance for the discus articularis but also compressive stress has its effect on the disk. This is particularly the case when the hand is in an ulnar abduction position, when stress is brought to bear on it (Arendt 1955). During ulnar abduction, the proximal carpal row of the hand moves in a radial direction and the os triquetrum comes into close contact with the discus articularis. Close joint contact is supposed to ensure transfer of the stress from the hand to the forearm. In numerous activities, as, for example, when pushing a heavy load, the hand is in ulnar abduction and most of the load is taken up by the root of the small finger (Von Baeyer 1930). With reference to the clear longitudinal movement of the two bones of the forearm during work with pneumatic machines, as observed by Laarmann (1956), Haage (1973) assumes that the distal shift of the caput ulnae must lead to a considerable compression of the discus articularis.

22

Movement of the caput ulnae of about 1.0–1.5 mm in a carpal direction, which causes compression of the discus articularis, can be demonstrated by roentgenography with healthy probands when the hand is pushed against an immovable object.

Morphological Evidence of Physiological Compressive Strain on the Disk. If it is assumed that the discus articularis not only fulfills the function of connecting and guiding the radius and ulna but also functions as a load-transferring element, then the question arises of to what extent this assumption is supported by morphological evidence. Studies carried out by Pauwels (1948, 1955, 1976) and Kummer (1956, 1959) portray spongy bone as rigid, trajectorial latticework. The spongiosa structure is similar to the normal stress trajectories in a homogeneous model subjected to pressure. If the spongiosa structure of the caput ulnae is examined in 2–3 mm thick transverse sections, roentgenograms show spongiosa running at right angles to the subchondral bone laminate and into the radial compacta of the neck of the ulna. These spongiosa bundles running into the subchondral compacta may be seen as pressure-absorbing elements (Fig. 17).

The fact that the caput ulna almost invariably has a cartilage surface layer that articulates with the discus articularis is a further indication of the transfer of compressive force. According to the principles of causal histogenesis (Pauwels 1960), articular cartilage is only retained in cases where compressive stress occurs with overlaid intermittent deformation.

The course of split lines on the articular sufaces of the caput ulnae and the os lunatum is characterized in each case by one attractive singular point. Attractive singular points indicate an articular surface that is subjected to considerable stress (Konermann 1971; Molzberger 1973; Tillmann 1978). In the os lunatum the point is situated dorsally in the ulnar region; in the caput ulnae it lies in a palmoradial position. These two areas are in line with each other through the intermediate disk when the hand is pronated and dorsally extended. When pressure is exerted, this is the normal position of the hand, and the radial part of the articular disk is compressed. The macroscopic observation that in adults the radial side of the disk is often rather thin, while in children the disk is uniformly thick, permits the conclusion that this side of the disk is affected in the long run by mechanical stress.

Histological examination of the disks from various age groups shows modification of the disk tissue. Whereas, in newborns and children the disk consists of close-knit bundles of collagen fibers and fibroblasts, with advancing age the central area comes to be composed mainly of cartilage cells. R. Fick (1904) described these cartilage cells without discussing their functional importance. Lang (1942), Arendt (1955), Hoegen and Reske (1956), Haage (1973), and Mikić (1978) see these cartilage cells as just one characteristic feature of a general degeneration process. Lang (1942) and Mikić (1978) compare visible features ("slimy spots, fatty degeneration, asbestos-like fiber decay, hyalinization of basic meterial," Lang 1942) with the changes that occur with age in other menisci or articular disks, as described by Tobler (1929), Niessen (1934), De Palma (1957), and Barnett et al. (1961).

According to Pauwels' view (1960) on the influence of mechanical stimuli on supporting tissue, the differentiation of hyaline cartilage presupposes primarily hydrostatic pressure. Hydrostatic pressure occurs in tissue when interior and exterior pressure is equal on all sides. Cartilage tissue is only retained when intermittent changes in form cause a kind of "kneading" ("Walkung," Pauwels 1960) of the tissue.

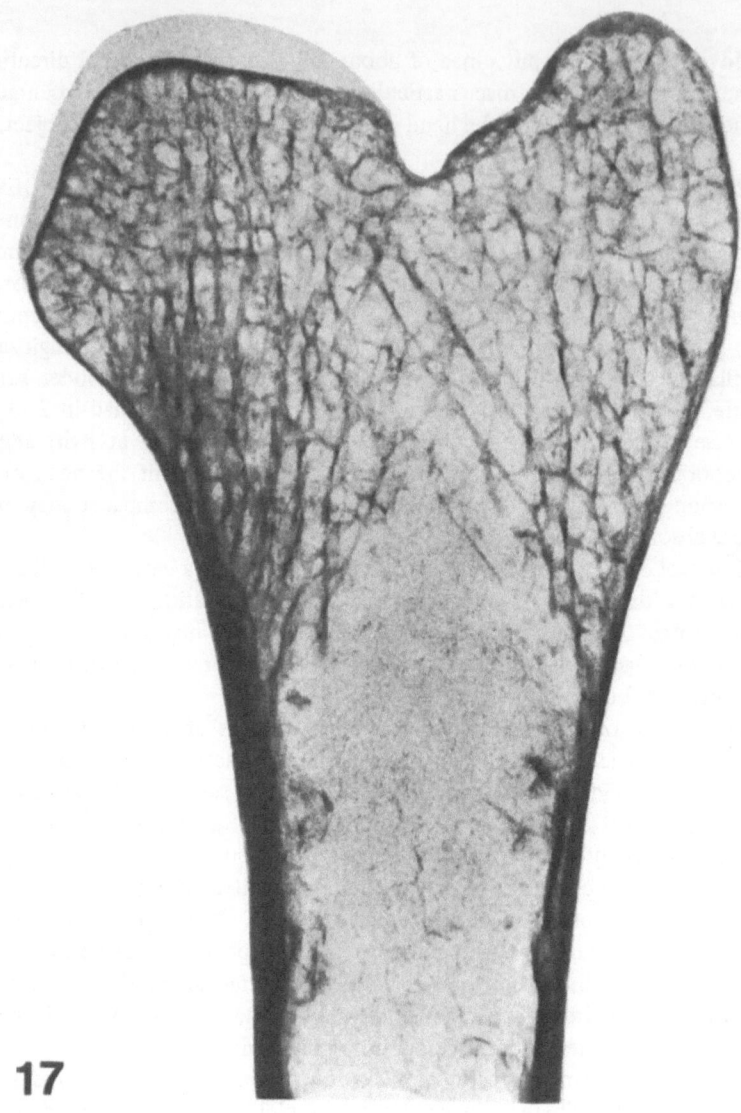

17

Fig. 17. Roentgenogram of a 2-mm-thick transverse section of the caput ulnae of an 80-year-old. Spongiosa radiates from the cartilage-covered distal articular surface into the radial compacta

Otherwise ossification occurs. The histological findings in the articular disk of the proximal wrist joint correlate with this process. Cartilage cells are seen to form in the center of the disk and intermittent deformation occurs due to compression of the disk between the caput ulnae and the os lunatum. From the theoretical viewpoint of causal histogenesis (Pauwels 1960), occasional cases of ossification are found to occur (Harris 1934; Köhler and Zimmer 1953; Thoms 1962) in the disk tissue in places where hydrostatic pressure prevails.

It has been shown that the described structural changes in the discus articularis correspond to normal physiological compressive stress. The development of cartilage cells demonstrates the functional adaptation of the tissue to compressive strain (Lang

24

1942; Arendt 1955; Mörike 1964). Particularly high mechanical load on the radial part of the disk leads to thinning of the tissue here, which ultimately results in the development of fissures or disk perforation. It is certainly possible that in individual cases not only the primary mechanical stress but also other factors may influence the structure of the disk, as remarked by Hoegen and Reske (1956). However, the main cause of changes in the disk structure must be seen to lie in mechanical compression of the disk due to its function.

Traumatic Lesion of the Disk. Traumatic lesions of the disk point to a single occasion of considerable compressive stress. Damage to the disk that occurs without fracture of the radius should be differentiated from lesions occurring together with or subsequent to a fracture of the radius in loco classico.

Disk Lesion Without Fracture of the Radius. Hoegen and Reske (1956) and Martinek (1977) report cases where bruising, spraining, or distortion of the proximal wrist joint resulted in a fissure, tear, or perforation of the discus articularis. Coleman (1960) reconstructed accidents and arrived at the conclusion that a disk lesion not accompanied by demage to the bone typically occurs when the hand is very extended in pronation. This corresponds to the results of this study with respect to the position of attractive singular points in the split line pattern and the occurrence of perforations in the radial part of the disk. When the hand is dorsally extended and pronated the os lunatum lies against the radial part of the disk. A simultaneous longitudinal force pushes the os lunatum into the disk like a wedge (Martinek 1977). If there is perforation of the disk over a large area, this also leads to incongruence of the articular surfaces of the caput ulnae and the os lunatum (Koebke and Brade 1980). This causes a decrease in the pressure-transmitting area and an increase in stress (cf. Pauwels 1961, 1963, 1968; Tillmann 1978); this is contrary to the view held by Mac Conaill (1931/32), who sees perforation of the disk as optimization of contact with the surface of the caput ulnae.

The incongruence leads to unphysiologically high strain on the articular cartilage. The morphological correlates of this excessive stress are found in the kind of localized cartilage deficiencies on the os lunatum and caput ulnae that Shepherd (1891) described.

Lesion Together with Classical Fracture of the Radius. In his study of classical fractures of the radius, Lang (1942) emphasizes the importance of the ulnar part of the proximal wrist joint. When classical fracture of the radius occurs, the discus articularis is either damaged at the same time, or posttraumatic changes are seen to take place. According to Lang (1942), Haage (1966), Rossak (1970), and Koebke and Brade (1980), the disk is subjected to extreme compression by the caput ulnae and the os lunatum when the radius is fractured. In addition to this compression, the disk is subjected to considerable traction when it is pulled taut over the caput ulnae as over a fulcrum, as the ulna is pushed towards the carpus by the force of impact.

Frykman (1967) commented on the inadequacies of comparable studies in the literature and carried out experiments to induce distal fractures of the upper limb. He showed that changes in the position of the hand lead to different kinds of fracture of the hand bones and the forearm. Classical fracture of the radius can be induced under static and dynamic conditions if the hand is in a position of $40°-90°$ of dorsal extension and $0°-35°$ of radial or ulnar abduction. Frykman's results allow him to

25

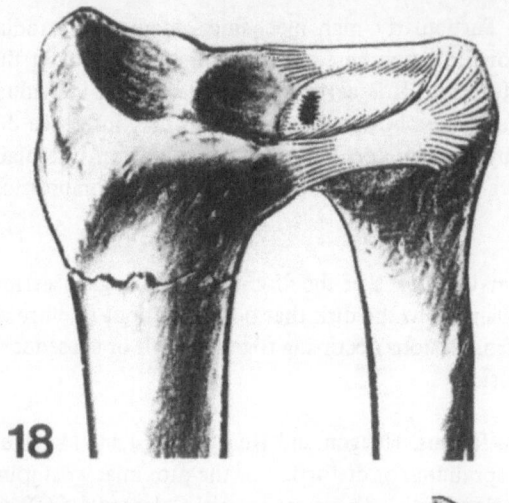

Fig. 18. Perforation of the discus articularis as a result of experimentally induced fracture of the radius

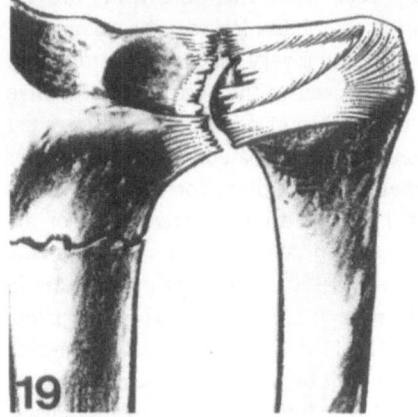

Fig. 19. Severance of the discus articularis as a result of experimentally induced fracture of the radius

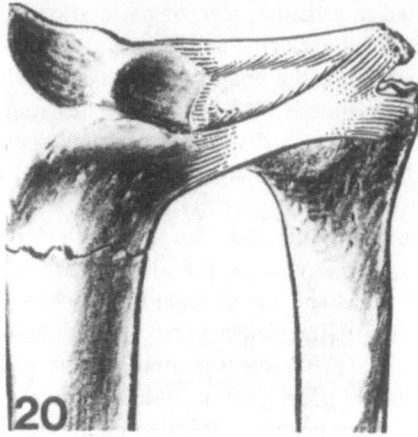

Fig. 20. Severance of the ulnar styloid process as a result of experimentally induced fracture of the radius. The disc itself is intact

classify distal fracture of the radius according to various criteria and to distinguish eight types of fracture. Experimentally induced distal fractures of the radius and the analysis of old radius fractures where the bone has knit together also permit conclusions to be drawn about the disk lesions that accompanied these fractures (Brade and Koebke in press). The disk may only show a fissure in the radial part, running in a dorsopalmar direction (Fig. 18). This has no effect on the function of the disk to connect radius and ulna. If the disk is completely ruptured at its radial fixation point (Fig. 19), the guidance and retention of the distal radioulnar joint is no longer ensured. Severance of the ulnar styloid process does not necessary involve a disk lesion (Fig. 20). However, if the disk also loses its second connection at the base of the styloid process, then joint contact between radius and ulna is ruptured. The ulna dislocates and protrudes toward the carpus (Fig. 21); this movement is assisted by the frequent development of a posttraumatically shortened radius (Lang 1942; Golden 1963; Böhler 1969; Pfeiffer et al. 1975; Martinek 1977; Küsswetter and Kibler 1977;

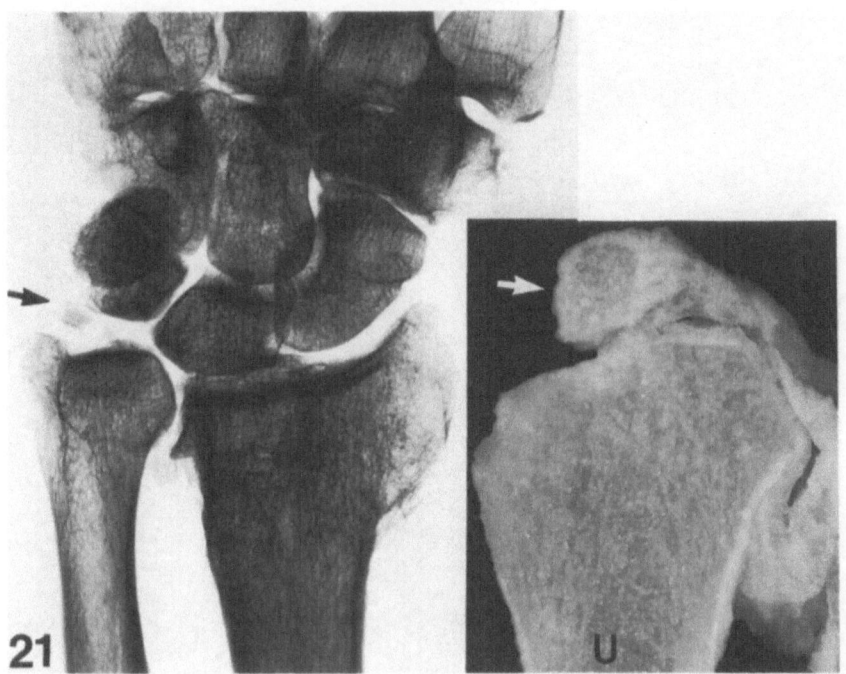

Fig. 21. Roentgenogram (PA) of a healed classical radius fracture (left arm of a 79-year-old woman). The ulna is in a distal position; the tip of the styloid process (→) is fractured. Osteophytic proliferations at the incisura ulnaris radii. Inset: Section through a similar fracture of the radius on the right arm of an 82-year-old man. The caput ulnae has moved in a distal direction, and the styloid process (→) has become separated

Poigenfürst and Tuchmann 1978). The resultant incongruence between the bones of the articulatio radioulnaris distalis leads to arthritic changes in the articular surfaces (Fig. 22).

Experimental Induction of Distal Fractures of the Radius and Load Effects on Radius and Ulna. As already mentioned, transfer of forces from the ulna to the radius via the membrana interossea antebrachii is often considered a factor contributing to fracture of the radius (Von Lanz and Wachsmuth 1959). Frykman's results (1967) lead him to doubt this theory, but he cannot disprove it because the arm preparations he used for his experiments consisted only of the hand and a distal section of the forearm. The results of the present study, on the other hand, which used arm preparations consisting of part of the humerus, the elbow joint, the entire forearm, and the hand, show that a classical fracture of the radius can also be induced when the membrana interossea has been severed. This is a clear indication that the membrane has no essential function as an energy transmitter. The experimental results show that the same kind of stress leads to fracture of the radius, irrespective of whether the membrana interossea is intact or not.

In contradiction to Mason's hypothesis (1954), in normal anatomic relations the radius and ulna are in contact with neighboring bones both in the articulatio cubiti and at the wrist joint. The discus articularis fills the gap between the caput ulnae

27

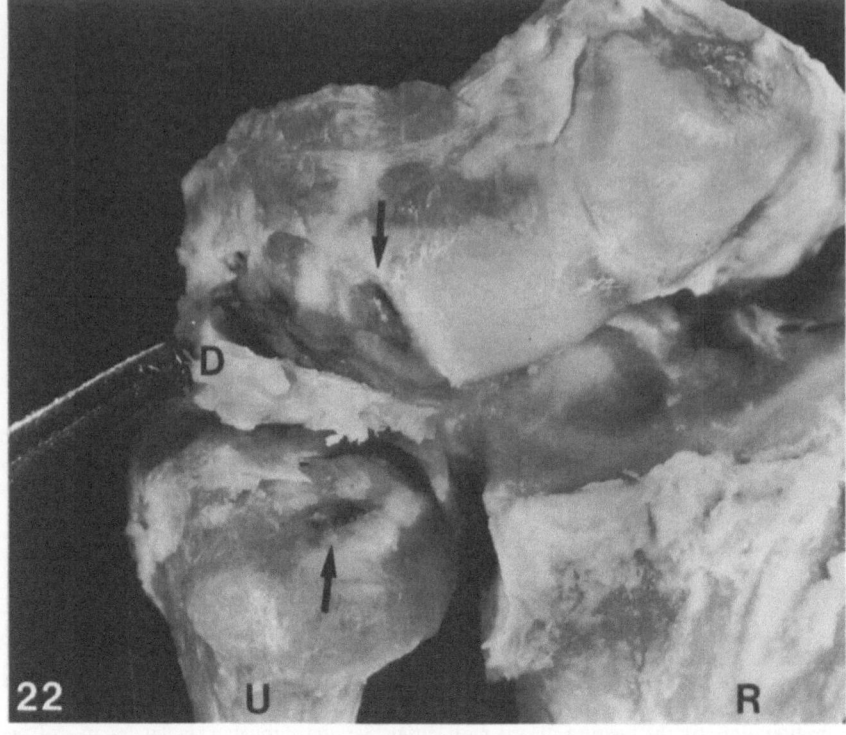

Fig. 22. Preparation of an old radius fracture (left arm of a 69-year-old man), dorsoulnar aspect. The disk (**D**) is completely ruptured at its radial fixation point (**R**, radius). The articular surfaces of the ulnar head (U) and the lunate show severe arthritic lesions (→)

and the os lunatum, functioning as a pressure-transmitting cushion. This means that stress transmitted from the upper arm to the forearm is taken up by both forearm bones.

The fact that stress often leads to fracture only of the radius can be explained by the disk acting as a shock absorber for the ulna. The stress on radius and ulna may also be unequal.

Transfer of Axial Load by the Radius and Ulna. Experiments carried out by Halls and Travill (1964) indicate that unequal stress transfer by radius and ulna is not dependent on force transmission by the membrana interossea. These authors used prepared ligamentous arms to measure the transfer of compressive forces in the elbow joint by exerting static pressure on the palm of the hand. The amount of pressure transferred by the radius to the capitulum humeri amounted, on average, to 57%. The ulna transmitted the remaining 43% to the trochlea of the humerus. The percentage relationship was not altered when the experiment was repeated after the membrana interossea had been severed.

The experimental method applied by these authors allows the definite conclusion to be drawn that the membrana interossea plays no essential role in the transfer of static forces. However, it appears doubtful whether the intraarticular measuring method used here permits exact data on the proportional transfer via radius and ulna, especially as the measuring gauges were not inserted under visual control. The authors give no information on the position of the elbow joint, the forearm bones, or the wrist joint.

Rossak (1965, 1970) measured the transfer of static pressure onto the two forearm bones by inserting a perspex capsule with resistance strain gauges into the two forearm bones of prepared arms and glueing them in below the membrana interoessea antebrachii. His results indicate that the proportional transfer of stress to the two forearm bones changes in connection with a change in the position of the forearm bones or the wrist joint. In a central or prone position when the hand is dorsally extended, almost all stress is transferred by the radius alone. In supination, 30%–50% of the pressure is transferred by the ulna. In arms where the membrana interossea had been severed, Rossak arrived at much the same results.

It should be noted, however, that the apparatus used by Rossak (1970) for his experiments – in particular, the stress frame holding the prepared forearm and the very local pressure transfer equipment – did not take important aspects of normal forearm load into consideration. Furthermore, it should be recalled, as indicated by Nikolic et al. (1975), that the occurrence of a classical fracture of the radius is always a dynamic and not a static matter.

In contrast to the methods described in the literature, the experimental method used in the present study to induce fractures and measure the transfer of kinetic energy simulates the effect of accelerated body weight during a fall onto the out-stretched hand at the moment of contact of the hand with the solid object. The kinetic energy is introduced to the arm *axially* via the stump of the humerus. The intact elbow joint is in an outstretched position. Carlsöö and Johansson (1962) show-ed that when a fall is stopped, the elbow joint is submitted almost exclusively to compressive strain. By embedding the hand, two aims are achieved: an equal counter-force affecting the thenar and hypothenar is simulated, and the position of the proxi-mal wrist joint can be precisely defined. By introducing kinetic energy to the forearm via the upper arm, it is possible to investigate the function of the membrana interossea antebrachii under dynamic load, which was not possible in the experiments carried out by Frykman (1967) and Nikolic et al. (1975).

The experimental results documented in this study show that when the hand is in a central or prone position, dorsally extended, and radially abduced, more than 80% of applied kinetic energy is transferred via the radius, irrespective of whether the membrana interossea is intact or not (Fig. 23). Increasing supination leads to an in-crease in the amount of stress taken up by the ulna, which may rise to up to 40%; with intact or severed membrane. In both pronation and supination, the amount of energy transferred by the radius is 3%–6% higher when the membrane has been severed than when it is intact (cf. Fig. 23). This permits the conclusion that when dynamic energy is transferred from the upper arm to the hand, the membrana interossea antebrachii is only importance to the value of 3%–6% of the energy.

There appear to be two possible reasons explaining the fact that in supination the proximal and distal transfer of kinetic energy to the ulna increases. Firstly, the action of supination means when the elbow joint is extended that the ulna comes to lie along the plane of load transfer, dictated in the experiment by the longitudinal axis of the humerus. Secondly, this tendency may be enhanced by adduction of the ulna to the radius during supination (Dwight 1885; Cathcart 1885; Heiberg 1885; Anderson 1901; Ray et al. 1951).

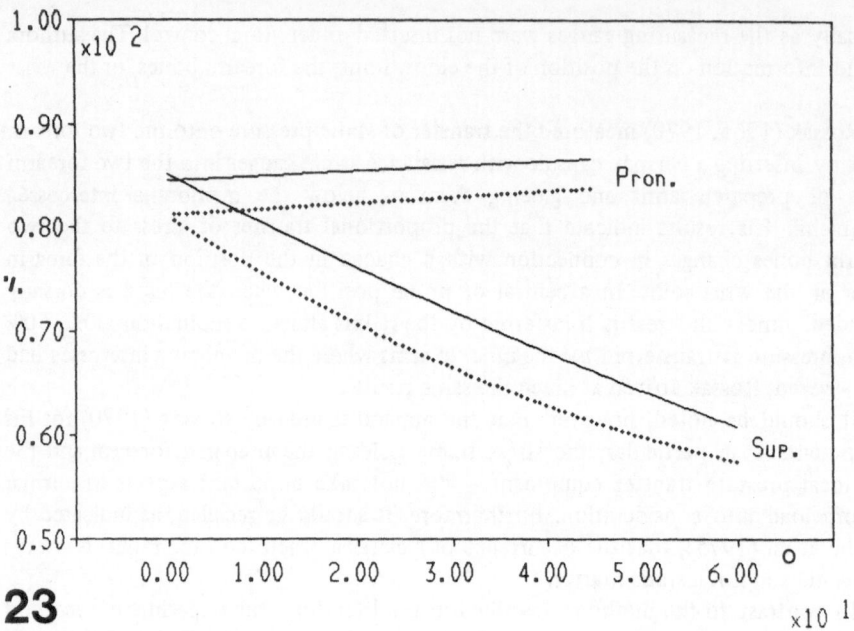

Fig. 23. Graph showing the kinetic energy transmitted by the radius when the membrana interossea antebrachii is intact (– – – –) and severed (————). When the membrane is severed, the amount of energy transferred by the radius increases in the neutral position, in pronation, and in supination by 3%–6%

This adduction means that the circumferentia articularis of the caput ulnae is pressed into the incisura ulnaris of the radius and held there. Contrary to the opinion expressed by R. Fick (1911), the adduction of the ulna is observed not only on living arms but also on dissected arm preparations (Vital et al. 1980).

It appears plausible to connect the adduction of the ulna with the membrana interossea, which is mostly taut during supination (Küsswetter 1979, 1981). Measurements obtained in the experiments discussed here imply that adduction still takes place when the membrane has been severed.

2.5 Conclusions

Results of this investigation may be summarized as follows: the membrana interossea antebrachii plays a very minor role in transferring kinetic energy from the upper arm to the hand. In a neutral position and in pronation, the radius is subjected to considerable strain. In this position the ulna is relatively little affected by the pressure exerted. With increasing supination, the amount of kinetic energy transferred by the ulna rises.

For the discus articularis situated between the proximal wrist joint and the caput ulnae, this means less compression during pronation and increasing compressive stress in supination, in both cases when the hand is dorsally extended. This obviously contradicts the findings from split line examination of the joint surfaces, but is explained by analyzing the use of the arm and the hand. Normally, the hand is not in a supinate position when under pressure load, but rather dorsally extended and in a prone position. The experimentally induced fracture of the radius is due to the immediate and extreme load brought to bear on the radius in pronation when the hand is dorsally extended and pressure applied. The strain transmitted by the ulna, although relatively small compared with that taken up by the radius, exceeds the physiological tolerance of the discus articularis. Lesions in the disk are the consequence.

The fact that falling onto the outstretched arm in pronation and dorsal extension often leads to a *distal* fracture of the radius is explained by Lewis (1950) and Rossak (1970) by a bending moment arising at this point. According to Rossak (1970), the bending force is due to traction from the volar capsule, which is taut during dorsal extension, and due to the volar intracapsular ligaments which, according to Taleisnik (1976) and Mayfield et al. (1976), are very strong.

Destot and Gallois (1896) suggest that the corticalis of the radius is particularly thin in the distal region and that is why a fracture often occurs here. However, the variation in the types of fracture documented in the clinical literature indicates, as also Böhler (1969) and Pfeiffer et al. (1975) among others believe, that in each individual case it is a combination of several factors that leads to the fracture at this particular point. In any case the single decisive factor, according to the results of the present study, is the extreme and direct compressive stress brought to bear on the radius.

3 Carpometacarpal Thumb Joint

3.1 Introduction

The importance of the thumb in connection with proper functioning of the hand as a whole is largely due to the particular morphology of the thumb's carpal joint. Unlike the other fingers, which are comparatively rigidly connected to the carpus, the articulatio carpometacarpea pollicis permits the thumb considerable. freedom of movement. The joint between the os metacarpale I and the os trapezium, referred to by Henke (1863) as the "purest" form of saddle joint, permits abduction and adduction of 35°–40° and flexion and extension of altogether 45°–60° (according to Fick 1911). These characteristic movements of the thumb take place around two axes (Fig. 24) situated at a 45° angle to the dorsopalmar and radioulnar carpometacarpal area (Fick 1854) and at right angles to each other, without traversing a common point. As shown by Toldt (1911), the abduction/adduction axis runs through the base of the first metacarpus, with the flexion/extension axis running in a radioulnar direction through the os trapezium.

Opposition of the thumb, which leads to the tip of the thumb being opposed to the tips of the other fingers, is a movement brought about not only by characteristic or basic thumb joint movements. Henke (1863) and Du Bois-Reymond (1895) showed the auxiliary movement in the thumb saddle joint necessary for opposition to take place. According to Meyer (1873) and Du Bois-Reymond (1896), this auxiliary movement is a purely axial rotation of the os metacarpale I. In contrast to this view, Bausenhardt (1949/50), Braus and Elze (1954), Napier (1955), Pieron (1973), and Kuczynski (1974) describe a circumductory movement of the first metacarpus that is

31

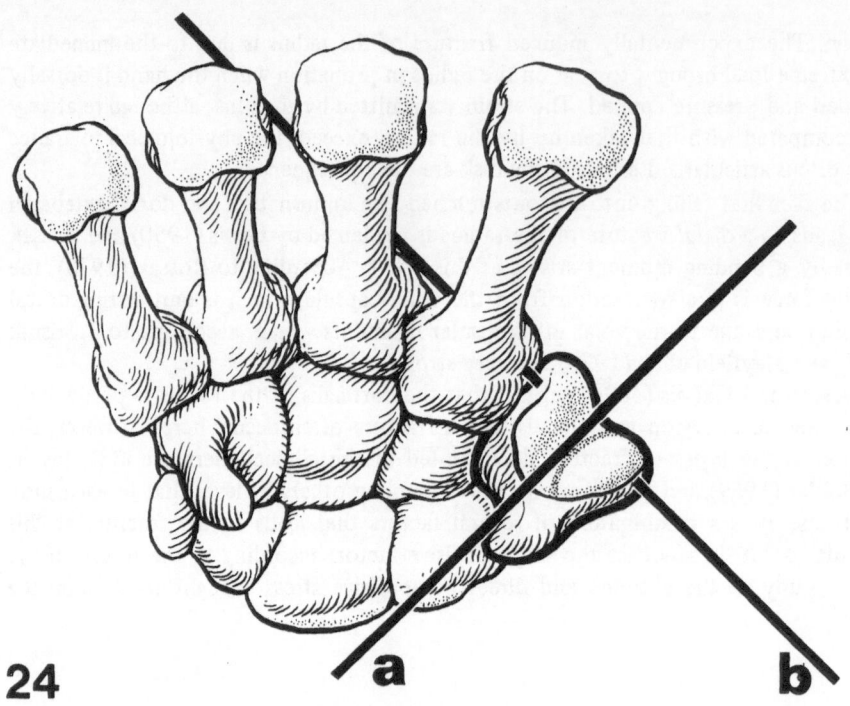

24   **a**   **b**

Fig. 24. Course of the two axes of the thumb saddle joint, around which the main movements take place. *a* abduction/adduction axis *b* flexion/extension axis

invariably combined with characteristic thumb joint movement and then leads to thumb opposition.

The articular surfaces of the thumb saddle joint may be compared with congruent, or almost congruent, silhouettes of geometrical figures. Bausenhardt (1949/50) "constructed" a swivel joint in which flexion of the thumb entailed rotation around the longitudinal thumb axis. Meyer (1873), however, considers the possibility of axial rotation of the thumb to be due to the fact the articulatio carpometacarpea pollicis is "really a very unclean joint." Considerable incongruence of the articular surfaces makes rotatory movement possible, activated by the m. opponens pollicis.

The incongruence of the articular surfaces has been confirmed by measurements, especially on the abduction/adduction level by Schmidt and Lieb (1981), but the question of how "unproblematic" rotatory movement between two saddle-shaped surfaces really is must still be considered an open issue. Von Lanz and Wachsmuth (1959) suggest that rotation is possible due to the malleable nature of the cartilage layer. According to Adler (1975), it is not only the flexibility of the cartilage but also the loose capsule that enable the thumb saddle joint to function as a ball-and-socket joint. Ligaments supporting the capsule are believed to induce the rotatory movement of the os metacarpale I (Fick 1911; Haines 1944; Bausenhardt 1949/50; Brown 1970; Pieron 1973; Landsmeer 1976).

According to Eaton and Littler (1969) and Kuczynski (1974), medial rotation of the os metacarpale I raises its saddle surface from the os trapezium. Thomas (1977) describes this movement as follows: the lower part of the saddle end of the os metacarpale I slides up on the side section of the higher saddle part of the os trapezium. In the final stage of this movement, partial contact of the articular surfaces takes place, with an increase in surface pressure. Pauwels (1963, 1968) notes that this kind of localized pressure area can be injurious to both bone and cartilage. The physiological rotation of the thumb saddle joint leads, according to Thomas (1977), to incongruent joint contact that may be regarded as "prearthrotic deformity" (Hackenbroch 1943), and can lead to arthrosis of the thumb saddle joint. The striking frequency of arthrosis of the thumb saddle joint (Bopp 1965; Bergk and Thümler 1979) has led in the literature to various interpretations of the etiology of this complaint (Müller 1949; Aune 1955; Cotta and Mittelmeier 1959; Schlegel 1965; Eaton and Littler 1969; Pfiffner 1971; Mannerfeld 1978; et al.).

The object of the present study is to investigate the extent to which primarily mechanical factors can lead to rhizarthrosis. The examination is based on adult hands from the dissection room. The following questions will be considered: 1. Are there morphological indications for (a) rotation in the thumb saddle joint in connection with opposition of the thumb, and (b) such rotation leading to incongruence of the articular surfaces?
2. Does articular incongruence lead to locally increased pressure and thus to cartilage damage?
3. Can split line pattern interpretation show whether the articular cartilage is suitably adapted to its functional role? Can the close examination of the capsule and the ligaments explain the abnormal joint position typical in advanced stages of rhizarthrosis?

3.2 Material and Methods

Sixty-eight left and right thumb saddle joints were examined; these came from hands dissected in a dissection course. The hands belonged to 21 male and 13 female corpses, aged between 25 and 96; only four of the subjects were under 50 years of age.

3.2.1 Roentgenographic, Equidensitometric, and Histological Examinations

Roentgenograms were made with all joints in about 25° pronation. In 20 of the thumb saddle joints, the muscles were removed and the capsule and ligaments analyzed. Particular attention was paid to the preparation and analysis of ligament connections between the base of the os metacarpale II and the capsule of the saddle joint. After the ligaments had been suitably prepared and photographed, the ligament connection point on the os metacarpale II and its line of connection to the joint capsule of the articulatio carpometacarpea pollicis were marked with the tip of a needle. New roentgenograms were then made to establish the position of the needle tips with respect to the metacarpal bones. The ligament was then severed at its point of connection with the joint capsule of the thumb saddle joint, but left intact where it joined with the os metacarpale II. By cutting a 2-mm thick bone section from this bone, the ligament was then isolated. Roentgenograms were also made of this ligament with its bone connection (Kodak, Definix Medical; 42 kV, 100 mAs).

The roentgenograms provide the primary data for exact quantitative evaluation of the density of bone tissue by means of a computerized television image analyzer (Schleicher et al. 1980). The X-ray film is placed between a slide and a glass slide cover and reduced to points by mechanical scanning. A picture analyzer determines the portion of each point that is not covered with particles of silver. This measuring method establishes the degree of exposure of the film. An aluminum scale included in the picture (Bergerhoff 1944) enables the values obtained to be quantified in terms of the corresponding X-ray-absorbing aluminum probe.

Finally, the ligaments are removed and used for histological examination. Sections 7–9 µm thick were stained with hematoxylin-eosin, azan, Goldner, resorcin-fuchsin van Gieson, and a calcium test according to Kossa.

3.2.2 Macroscopic Examination, Production of Split Lines, and Photoelastic Experiments

On 48 hands, the muscles were removed and the joint capsule laid free, the joint opened, and the articular surfaces macroscopically examined and photographed. Localization and extent of cartilage deficiencies of both articular surfaces were determined with the aid of a magnifying glass and noted in the photographs. Loose bodies in the joint were isolated and decalcified in EDTA solution prior to further histological examination. The same procedure was applied in the case of five degenerated ossa trapezia, together with their respective base parts of the metacarpal bone.

Production and evaluation of split line patterns was done according to Konermann's method (1971; see Sect. 2.2.2).

Photoelastic Experiments. The general physical principles of the photoelastic method have been set out in detail by Föppl and Mönch (1950), Kummer (1959), and Knief (1967). Stress distribution on the articular surfaces of the articulatio carpometacarpea pollicis was analyzed with the help of two-dimensional models made of a type of plastic characterized by double breaking under stress (PV 1527, 10 mm thick). The models were subjected to equal, even stress in a metal frame and placed between the polarized light source and analyzer of a special photoelastic apparatus. The isochromes that became visible under stress in polarized light were photographed. When white, circular polarized light is used, the isochromes indicating points of equal stress difference are re-presented as bands of the same color. The colored isochrome bands show up as black when a red filter is used. The consecutive number of a given isochrome can be seen as a relative measure of the degree of stress difference at a given point on the model (Kummer 1959).

3.3 Results

3.3.1 Results from Roentgenography and Macroscopic and Split Line Examinations

Of the 68 thumb saddle joints examined, 30 showed signs of degenerative arthritic change, as seen from the roentgenograms. There were 6 cases with slight narrowing of the joint cleft and slight, localized sclerosis of the subchondral bone, while 24 further cases were found to show pronounced defects with loss of the joint cleft, de-formation of the articular surfaces, and thickening of the subchondral bone (Fig. 25a). Pseudocysts were only found in the os trapezium. In 12 of these 24 cases, uncovered bone was found on the articular surface in places. In five cases, there was clear radial subluxation (Fig. 25b) of the metacarpal thumb bone on the os trapezium. Of the other 38 thumb joints, 29 showed no pathological degeneration on the X-ray films. Three joints gave evidence of decay corresponding macroscopically to primary chronic polyarthritis. In four arthritic joints and three that were roentgenographically normal, a small spur of bone was found at the base of the os metacarpale II on the radial side (Fig. 25c).

All 20 prepared joints showed a ligamentous connection between the base of the os metacarpale II and the thumb saddle joint capsule. The ligament was anchored at

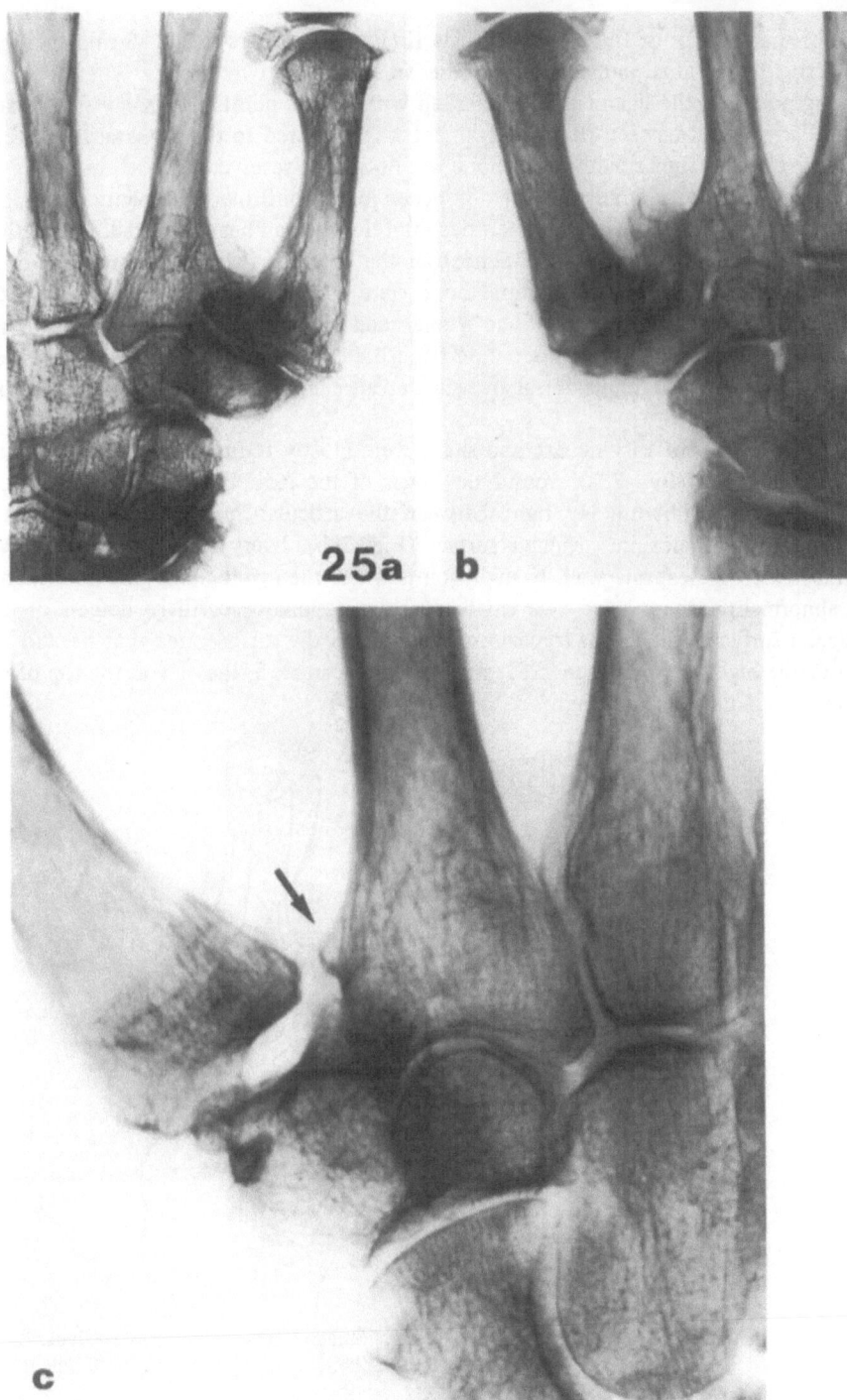

Fig. 25. *a* Roentgenogram of a rhizarthrosis on the left hand of an 83-year-old woman; narrow joint cleft, sclerosis of the subchondral bone, and osteophytic proliferations. *b* Roentgenogram of a rhizarthrosis on the left hand of a 66-year-old woman. Radial subluxation of the first metacarpal bone. *c* Spur of bone (*arrow*) at the radial base of the os metacarpale II on the left hand of a 51-year-old man

the dorsoradial base of the os metacarpale II (Fig. 26), where it is 2–5 mm thick. It ran across to the ulnarpalmar joint capsule, frequently in two strands. When the connecting points of the ligament were marked with needle points and X-ray films made (Fig. 27), it could be seen that the ligament was anchored to the os metacarpale II at the very place where a small spur of bone was noticed in seven cases.

Macroscopic examination of the 48 opened joints confirmed the roentgenographic findings in all 26 cases where degenerative joint defects had been detected. In addition to finding articular surfaces were almost all the cartilage had disappeared and clear signs of abrasion on the subchondral bone were apparent, in ten cases the os metacarpale I and the os trapezium had a one-sided palmar area[4] where there was no cartilage. This area was clearly separate from the cartilage-covered dorsal part. In all these cases, the cartilaginous dorsal area showed a small, local defect on the metacarpal side.

Loose bodies of varying size and shape were mostly found in the palmar or ulnar part of the joint (Fig. 28a) around the edges of the joint capsule. In two cases, a spherical corpus liberum lay right between the articular surfaces, embedded in a hollow in the trapezium articular surface (Fig. 28b). Every loose body found was connected to the capsule wall. In eight joints where roentgenograms gave no evidence of abnormality, there were two small local depressions or cartilage defects on the articular surfaces. On the os trapezium, these lay in the surface area that rises to the top of the high part of the saddle; on the os metacarpale I, they lay at the top of the proximal saddle arm (Fig. 28c).

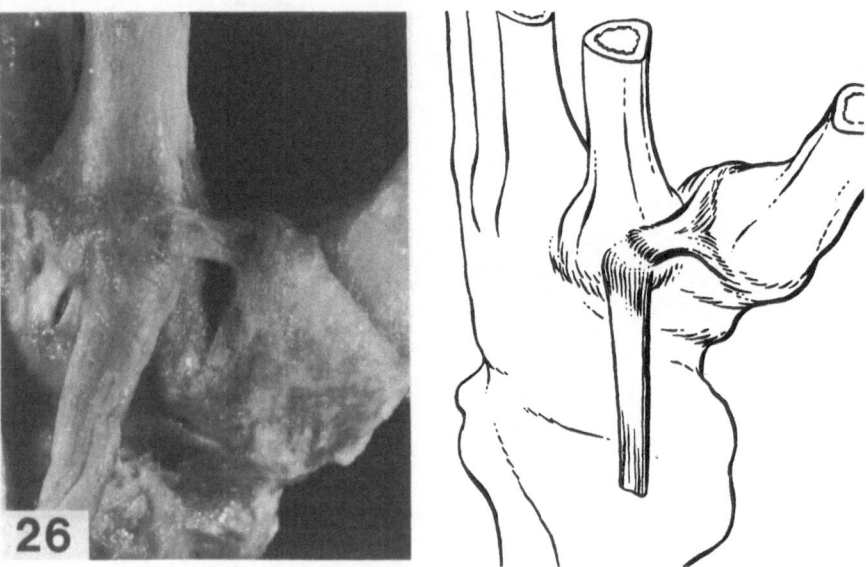

Fig. 26. Preparation (*left*) and drawing (*right*) of the ligament between the os metacarpale II and the capsule of the thumb saddle joint. Dorsal view left, dorsoradial view right. The ligament is in two strands where it enters the joint capsule

---

[4] Descriptions of position and direction refer to a basic position in which the thumb saddle joint lies as the other carpometacarpal joints do. The two main joint axes are then dorsopalmar (abduction/adduction axis) and radioulnar (flexion/extension axis).

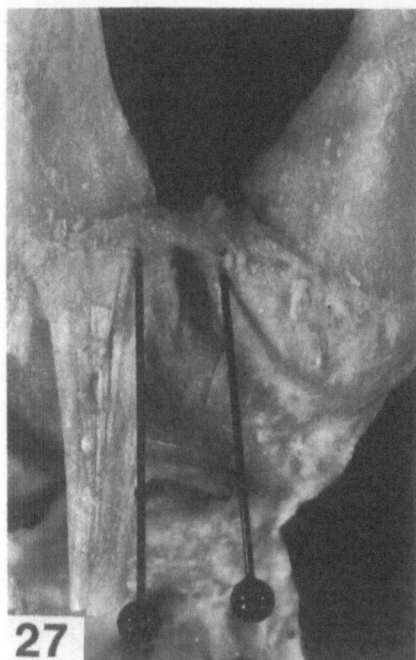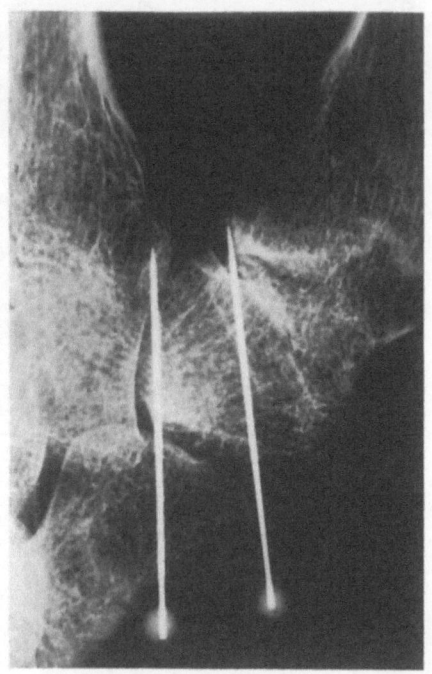

Fig. 27. Ligament insertions marked by metal pins on prepared material (*left*) and on roentgenogram (*right*). The left needle tip lies at the radial base of the os metacarpale II

Split Line Pattern of Os Metacarpale I. Split lines were found to run in identical patterns on 14 normal metacarpal articular surfaces as well as on the eight that showed small depressions. In the central area, the lines ran parallel to each other from the lower dorsal to the lower palmar side of the saddle. The lines deviated increasingly towards the ulnar and radial higher side of the saddle, with a radial and an ulnar attractive singular point (Fig. 29a).

Split Line Pattern of the Os Trapezium. The split line pattern of the trapezium articular surfaces examined here was less uniform. In 12 ossa trapezia, where the articular surface was almost square, there were four bow-shaped lines arising from the peripheral articular surface (Fig. 29b) and describing an arch back to back against a central repulsive singular point. Where the articular surface was more triangular (in eight cases), there were three such bow-shaped lines (Fig. 29c), again around a repulsive singular point. A pattern variant that was observed in two cases had, in addition to the four lines from the corners, a bow-shaped line stemming from the lower dorsal side of the saddle and containing a central attractive singular point. The palmar and ulnar articular surface areas had one repulsive singular point each.

3.3.2 Photoelastic Findings

The two-dimensional plastic models and the articular surfaces they represent corresponded to frontal sections of the two bones of the saddle joint. In the first

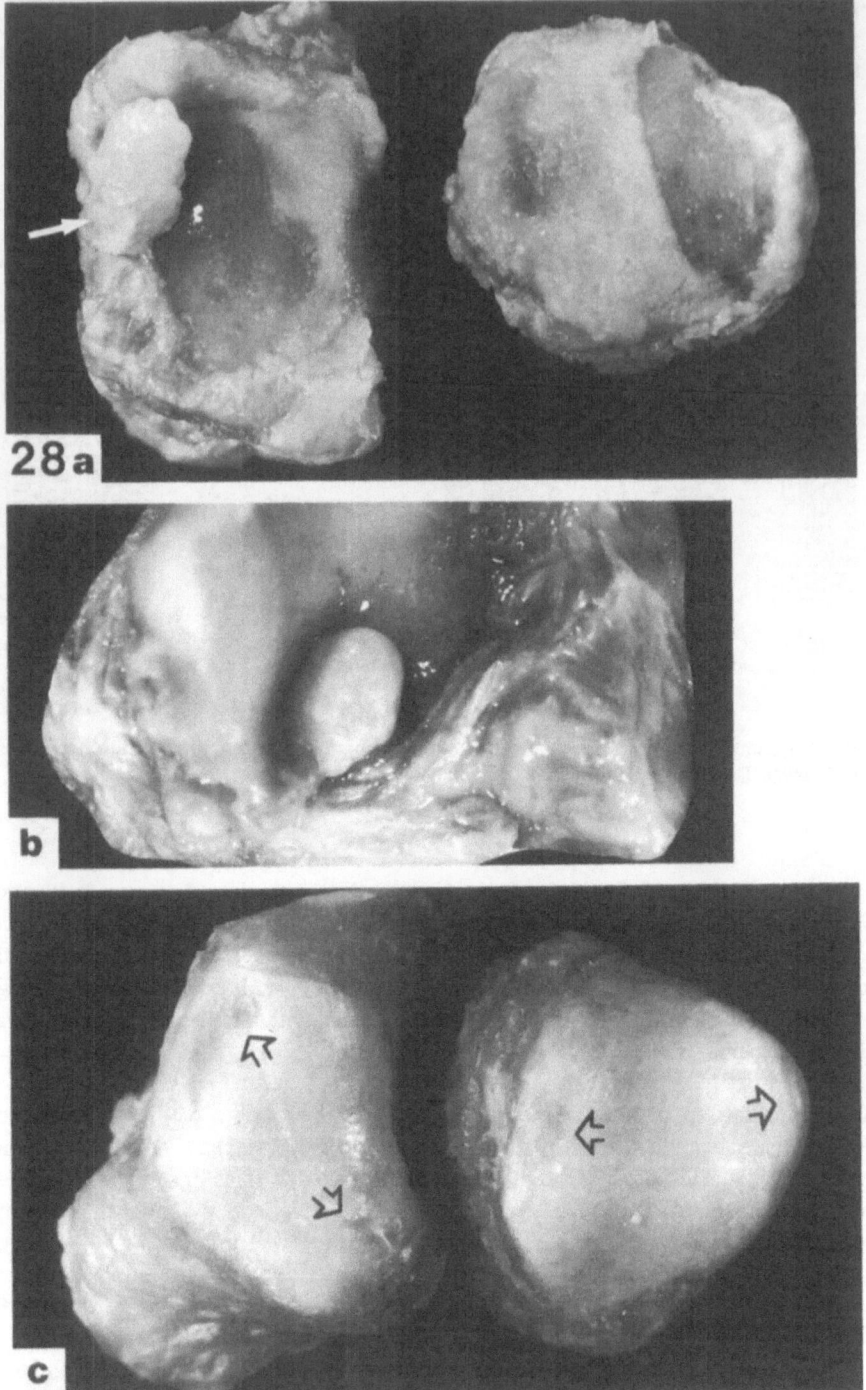

Fig. 28. *a* Articular surfaces of the right saddle joint of a 67-year-old woman. The palmar areas of the metacarpal (*right*) and trapezial (*left*) surfaces are free of cartilage. A loose body (*arrow*) lies at the palmar edge of the os trapezium. *b* Large corpus liberum embedded in the right os trapezium of a 73-year-old man. *c* Right opened saddle joint of a 51-year-old woman with local depressions (*arrows*) at the trapezial (*left*) and metacarpal (*right*) surfaces. (*a* and *c* from Koebke and Thomas 1979a)

38

experiment, a joint model representing the two articulating members in congruent position was subjected to pressure. In this case, the base of the os metacarpale I was convex and the surface of the os trapezium concave. Isochromes were almost symmetric in both halves of the joint model. The isochrome with the consecutive number, 0, lay on the edge of the model sections, and the isochrome with the highest consecutive number, 3, in the central part (Fig. 29d).

In the second experiment, the contact between the two halves of the model corresponded to the articulation between the os metacarpale I and the os trapezium after ulnar rotation of the thumb. In this position the model was subjected to even pressure, as in the first experiment. Particular areas of stress were observed in the contact zones; the last still clearly discernible isochromes were numbers 7 and 8 (Fig. 29e).

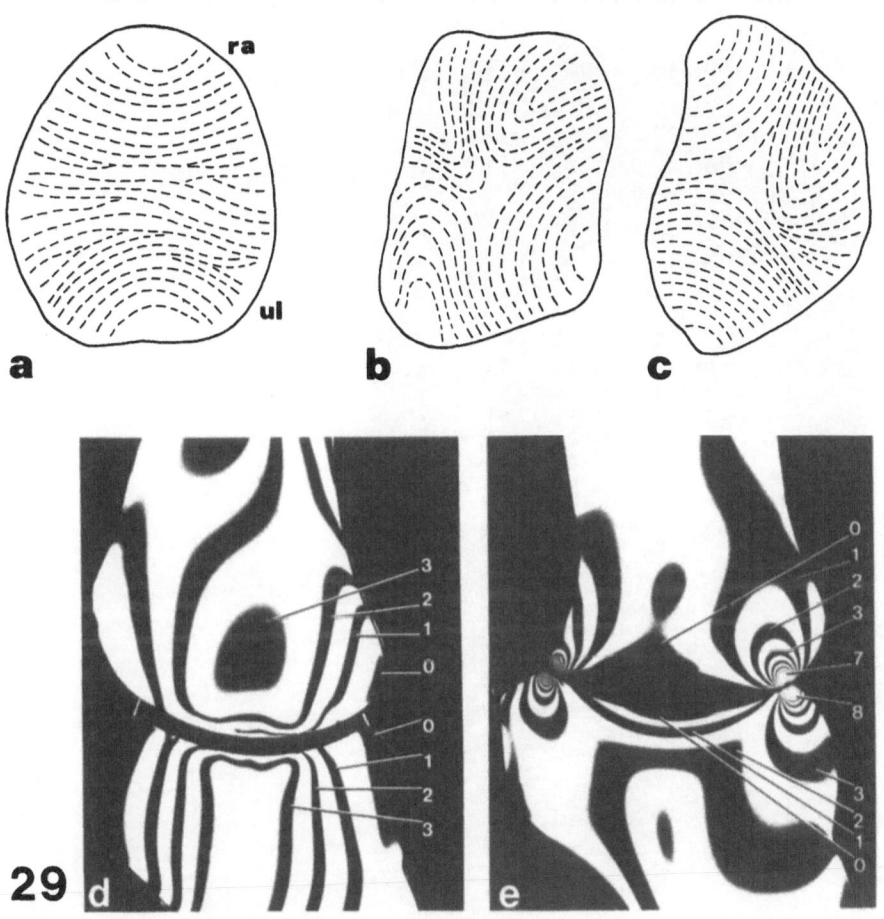

Fig. 29. Split lines on the articular surfaces of the thumb saddle joint: *a* basic pattern on the metacarpal articular surface (*ra*, radial, *ul*, ulnar); *b* split lines on an almost rectangular trapezial surface; *c* split lines on a triangular-oval trapezial articular surface. *d* Stress distribution in a model of the saddle joint with congruent position of the os metacarpale I upon the os trapezium. The isochromes are symmetric. *e* High local stresses in a model of the incongruent saddle joint with reduced contact zones. (*d* and *e* from Koebke and Thomas 1979a)

3.3.3 Density Measurements and Histological Findings

In 6 of the 20 prepared ligaments, patches of thickening in the ligamentum meta-carpeum dorsale I could be seen on the roentgenograms. These patches lay in the ulnar part of the ligament where it approaches the os metacarpale II (Fig. 30a).

Quantitative analysis by the equidensity method showed these patches of thickening to be a clearly defined zone, corresponding to an aluminum equivalent 0.5–1 mm thick (Fig. 30b). Histological examination of the ligament in cross sections and longitudinal sections showed bundles of collagen fibers, mainly in a longitudinal direction. A few elastic fibers could be observed. In these six cases, there were fine- to coarse-grained calcium deposits in the ulnar part of the ligament near the connection to the os metacarpale II (Fig. 31).

Histological examination of the isolated corpora libera produced a variety of findings. Three of them consisted of fibrous tissue containing chondroid cells. They

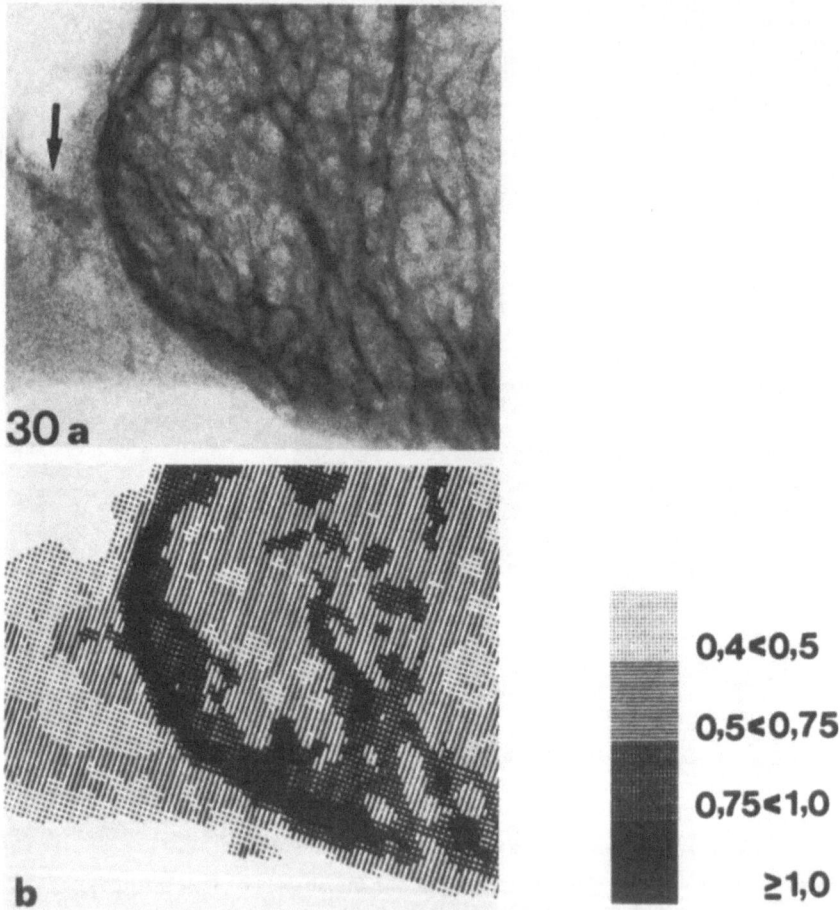

30 a

b

0,4<0,5

0,5<0,75

0,75<1,0

≥1,0

Fig. 30. Calcification of the ligamentum metacarpeum dorsale I: *a* Calcification visible on roent-genogram (*arrow*) within the ligament near the base of the os metacarpale II. Section 2 mm thick. *b* Equidensity picture of the same section with ligament. Zone of calcification corresponds to 0.5–1.0 mm aluminum

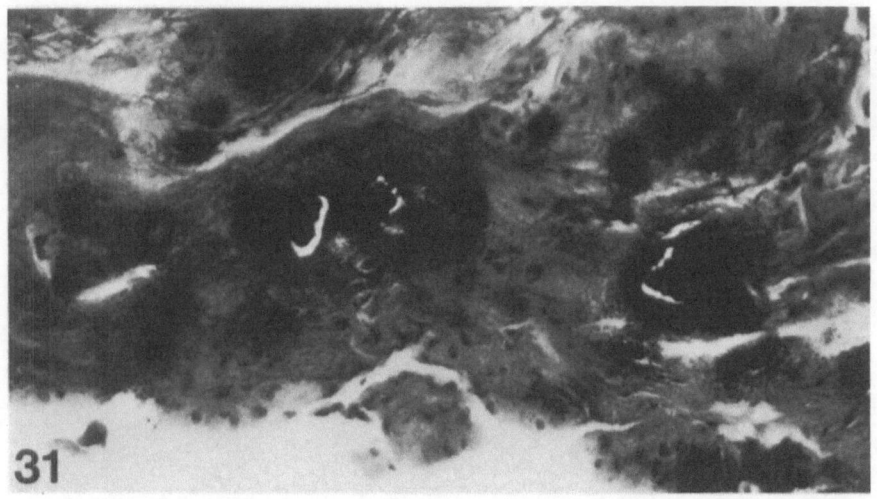

Fig. 31. Histological longitudinal section through the ulnar part of a ligamentum metacarpeum dorsale I with granular calcium deposits. Kossa, 8 μm; × 56

were connected to the membrana fibrosa of the joint capsule by way of numerous dense collagen fibers. The capsule tissue itself was vascular. The other bodies in the joint capsule had a central nucleus composed of bone tissue, surrounded by a layer of fibrous tissue of varying thickness. Within this fibrous tissue, there were isolated patches of hyaline cartilage. Two smooth-topped corpora libera, lying embedded in the os trapezium, were found to have a tissue coating that was relatively thick in comparison with the bone tissue nucleus, and that was composed of layers (Fig. 32; cf. Fig. 28). Next to the exterior membrana synovialis was a thin layer of dense connective tissue, which gave way to a layer of hyaline cartilage tissue with some fibers. The next layer then consisted of fibrous cartilage of about the same thickness, which surrounded the central nucleus of bone tissue.

The cartilage of degenerated articular surfaces of the os trapezium and os metacarpale I was found to be coarse and roughly fibrous on the surface in some places. Occasionally there was no cartilage layer left, so that the subchondral bone showed through, showing signs of sclerosis.

3.4 Discussion

Morphology and Articular Mechanism of the Articulatio Sellaris. The fact that the thumb can be brought into the position known as opposition, whereby the thumb can "make a fist in contact with every finger" (Fick 1911), is largely due to the particular shape of the articular members of the articulatio carpometacarpea pollicis. A. Fick (1854), who suggested the use of the term saddle joint to describe this joint, investigated the geometry of articular surfaces and the movements involved. Having observed that the articular surfaces have a corresponding and reciprocal curvature, he compared the joint members with a one-sheet hyperboloid of rotation. Geometrical surfaces with characteristics similar to A. Fick's hyperbolic function and "negative" also formed the

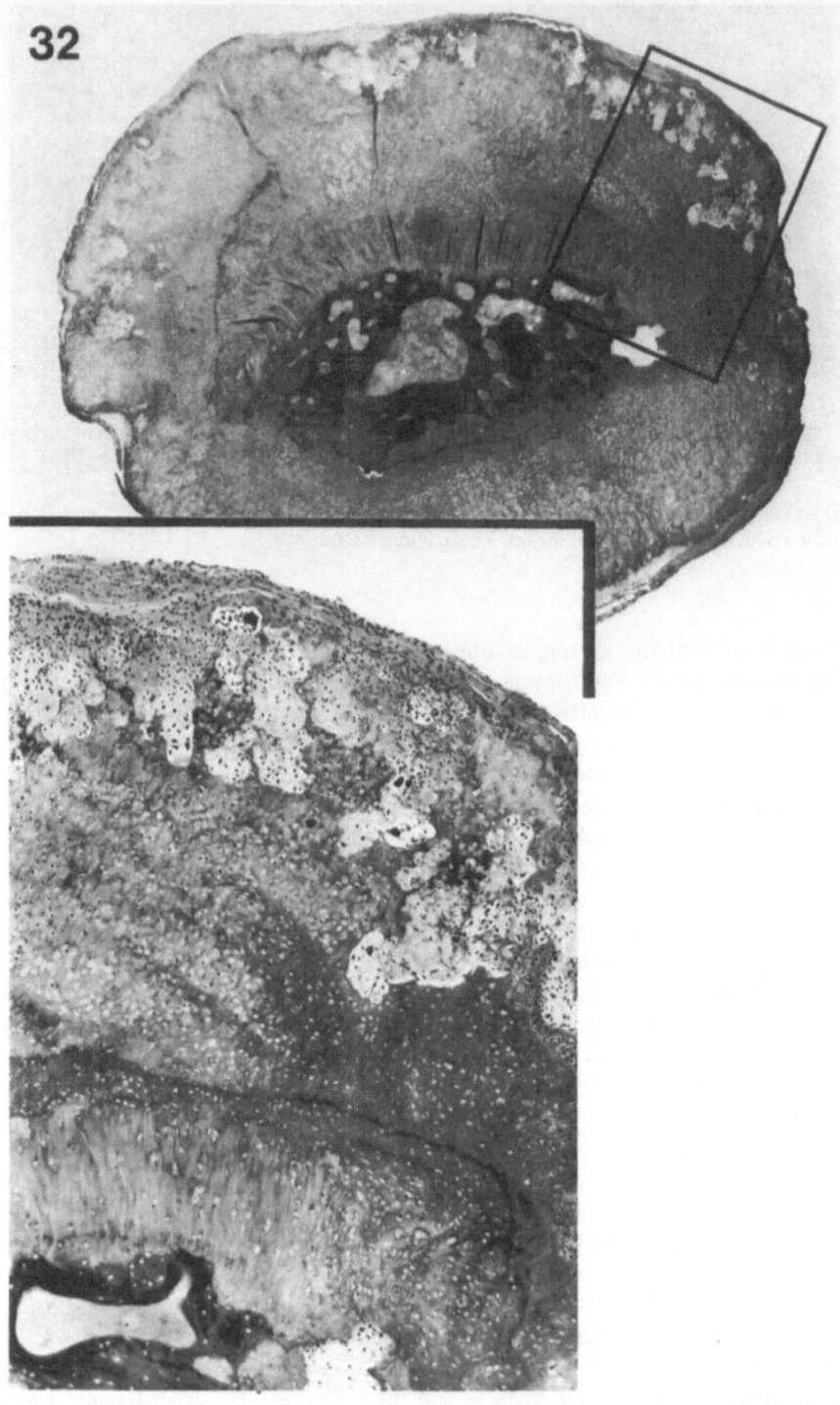

Fig. 32. Corpus liberum with smooth surface and layered structure. The exterior membrana synovialis is next to a thin layer of collagen fibers; next is a thin layer of hyaline cartilage that gives way to fibrous cartilage. This continues to the core of bone. Azan, 10 μm; × 18, inset × 57

basis for Henke's (1863) hypothesis. He was able to show that surface segments of two interlocking touching circular rings of the same size and curvature are congruent saddle areas. Meyer (1873) defined the articulatio carpometacarpea pollicis as a ginglymus with saddle-shaped articular surfaces. All these geometrically based joint forms are, as remarked on by Du Bois-Reymond (1895), restricted to two axes for their scope of movement. One traverses the os trapezium (flexion/extension axis), the other runs dorsopalmarly through the base of the os metacarpale I (abduction/adduction axis). According to Du Bois-Reymond (1896), strict adherence to Fick's (1854) geometric model of the hyperboloid of rotation excludes one of the two theoretically possible movements, so that hinged movement is possible around only one axis. In the case of two connecting congruent torus segments, there will be increasing dehiscence, at least during movement around one of the two axes.

Because of the obvious deficiencies of all previous models, Du Bois-Reymond (1896) developed what he considered to be "the theoretically most perfect type of saddle joint": if the same degree of congruent movement about two axes is to be possible between two saddle joints, then both axes must be on one level. The two joint members should only meet at the crossing-point of the two axes and otherwise, as they have curved surfaces, should roll freely on each other. This necessitates a more convex and a concave surface. According to Du Bois-Reymond's curvature measurements, this prerequisite is fulfilled. The convex curvature of the os trapezium corresponds to an arc from a circle with an 8-mm radius, and the concavity of the os metacarpale I is that of a circle with a 12.5-mm radius. The concave surface on the os trapezium was measured to be 18 mm, while the radius of the convex curvature of the os metacarpale I was 12.5 mm. These findings of Du Bois-Reymond (1896) must be compared with those of Günther (1850), who found almost the same values for the reciprocal curve profiles of the os trapezium and os metacarpale I. R. Fick (1904) doubts the validity of the measurements of the two authors, largely because the test population was too small; for example, Du Bois-Reymond's measurements were based on only 13 joints.

Schmidt and Lieb (1981) examined the articular surfaces of the same two bones in 150 cases, some of which were macerated. They were able to show that the curvature radius of the os trapezium in the radioulnar direction (level of abduction/adduction is always greater than that of the corresponding os metacarpale. However, curvatures found were not always basically circular, but also spiral or S-shaped. This confirms the hypothesis previously made by Meyer (1873), Fischer (1897), and R. Fick (1904), who maintained that the articular surfaces of the thumb saddle joint do not correspond to sections of perfect geometric rotary bodies but only to approximations of these. The fact that more recent theoretical discussions by Kapandji (1963), Duparc et al. (1971), Kapandji (1972), and Dahhan et al. (1980) ignore this issue does not make their content any more valid, especially as familiar rotary bodies (hyperboloid of rotation, torus) also form the basis of their considerations. Describing the articulatio carpometacarpea pollicis as a universal joint (Kapandji 1972; Dahhan et al. (1980) does not account for morphological facts.

Rotational Movement of the Thumb Saddle Joint. The observation that opposition of the thumb entails not only the main movements around the curved surfaces but also rotation was made early by Henke (1863) and Du Bois-Reymond (1895). The latter determined the total rotation of the thumb by measuring the change in direction of small pins inserted on the surface. He measured medial rotation of the thumb up to 30°. His conception of the model of a saddle joint with differing concave and convex curvature radii of the joint bones allows for rotary movement, which always occurs together with flexion.

In addition to this, Du Bois-Reymond maintains there is 30° rotation in the metacarpophalangeal joint. This value is much higher than those postulated by Duchenne (1867), Strasser (1917), and Braus and Elze (1954), and his own measurements led Kaplan (1966) to doubt it. Meyer (1873) discounted the possibility of rotation in the metacarpophalangeal joint of the thumb but supported the hypothesis that there is rotation of the os metacarpale I in the thumb saddle joint. His functional analysis of the muscles of the thumb divided muscles into those responsible for abduction and adduction, for flexion and extension, and for opposition and reduction. He considered opposition and reduction to be those rotary movements which cause the radial edge of the thumb metacarpus to move towards or from the vola manus. R. Fick (1904), on the other hand, considered movements of opposition and reposition to be identical to the flexion/extension movements in the thumb saddle joint around the radioulnar axis.

The definition that goes back to A. Fick (1854), which is also the most common one in modern anatomic textbooks, does not take rotary movement into account. Rotation is seen as a compulsory accessory movement. Bunnel (1938) correctly remarked that simple flexion (or opposition, according to Fick's definition) in the articulatio carpometacarpea pollicis does not lead to opposition, in the sense that the thumb tip is diametrically opposite the finger tip of one of the other fingers. Napier (1955, 1956) also saw opposition as a complex movement in the thumb saddle joint that includes a component of rotation. This view was supported by Bausenhardt (1949/50), Landsmeer (1962), Eaton and Littler (1969), Kuczynski (1974), Bojsen-Møller (1976), Thomas (1977), Koebke and Thomas (1979a, 1979b), and Guyot (1981).

In spite of varying definitions for opposition, it is clear that rotary movement does take place in the thumb saddle joint. This occurs in combination with other movements. The question of the extent to which the shape of the joint members facilitates rotary movement of the metacarpus is not viewed in the same light by all scientists. Fick (1904), Fischer (1919), Grünkorn (1932), and Von Lanz and Wachsmuth (1959) all indicate the cartilage layer to be about 1 mm thick, which they consider rather thick. They see its deformability as neccessary for rotation in the saddle joint. However, it should be recalled that a certain degree of deformability is a typical characteristic of hyaline cartilage (Pauwels 1960; Kummer 1975; Oberländer 1978). In view of results obtained by Stümpel and Koebke (in press), it appears doubtful whether the cartilage layer on the articular surfaces of the articulatio carpometacarpea pollicis is really to be considered particularly thick. As a point of comparison, the cartilage of the metacarpophalangeal joints II–V is up to 1.3 mm thick.

Bausenhardt (1949/1950) developed the model of a modified ball-and-socket joint for the thumb saddle joint. He considered the articular surface of the os trapezium to represent approximately half of a one-sheet hyperboloid of rotation. During oppositional movement, the os metacarpale I slides congruently in the bowl of the rotary body. At the same time, the turning metacarpus rotates around the axis of the hyperboloid. Because the convex curvature of the os metacarpale I has a smaller radius than the reciprocal concave profile of the os trapezium, abduction and adduction can take place as a combined roll-and-slide movement. Napier (1955) and Ramselaar (1970) based their deliberations on the highly convex curvature of the metacarpal articular surface. Starting from an incongruent central position, where the metacarpus is only in contact with the os trapezium on one point in the abduction/adduction plane, abduction of the thumb takes place. In the abduction position, the joint cleft is apparent in a dorsoulnar direction and the second step is then opposition when the os metacarpale I describes a circumductory movement towards the palm of the hand. In this second phase of a so-called diadochal movement, axial rotation is conjunct, according to Mac Connaill (1946).

Apart from this indirect explanation of opposition that applies when large objects are to be held in the hand, Napier (1955) and Ramselaar (1970) considered another, more direct form of opposition. From the incongruent central position, they maintain that medial rotation of the os metacarpale I can be combined with flexion and abduction, for example, when taking hold of a small object between thumb and index finger. Pieron (1973) also described a circumductory movement of the os metacarpale I from the position of abduction, possible because of the incongruency of the articular surfaces. However, he maintained that circumduction in oppositional movement describes a longer trajectory than in reposition.

Loss of Articular Surface Congruency. An observation that has a bearing on the results of the present study was made by Kuczynski (1974). He described how the passively opposed os metacarpale I was twisted out of the saddle of the os trapezium in prepared, amputated material. He considered it likely that the same applied to active movement in opposition and reposition of the living hand. Support for the hypothesis is provided by the results of similar examinations by cinematographic roentgenograms of living people carried out by Eaton and Littler (1969).

Incongruence of the Thumb Saddle Joint as a Prearthritic Deformity. Thomas (1977) based his hypothesis concerning the development of arthrosis in the thumb saddle joint on the movement that twists the metacarpal articular surface out of the saddle of the os trapezium during opposition. He believed that rotation in the articulatio carpometacarpea pollicis leads to incongruence in the joint, with only partial contact of the articular surfaces. The low saddle arms of the metacarpal surface glide onto the high part of the trapezial saddle, and load is transferred via reduced surfaces and, therefore, under increased pressure. Thomas saw the loss of articular surface congruency as a prearthritic deformity in the sense implied by Hackenbroch (1943).

Cartilage Defects as a Morphological Correlate of Physiological Incongruency. In some cases where roentgenograms showed normal, intact joints, there were found to be local hollows or pinhead-sized defects in the cartilage surface. These lay close to the tip of the low saddle arms of the os metacarpale I (concave curvature) and to the tip of the high part of the articular saddle surface of the os trapezium (convex curvature, Fig. 33a; cf. Fig. 28c).

The small cartilage lesions are a morphological indication of the rotation taking place in the thumb saddle joint. If the thumb of a prepared joint is placed in opposition, the base of the metacarpus is automatically twisted out of the saddle of the os trapezium (Fig. 33b). This "sliding up" of the saddle arm takes place both when the joint is in a central position and when it is in abduction.

45

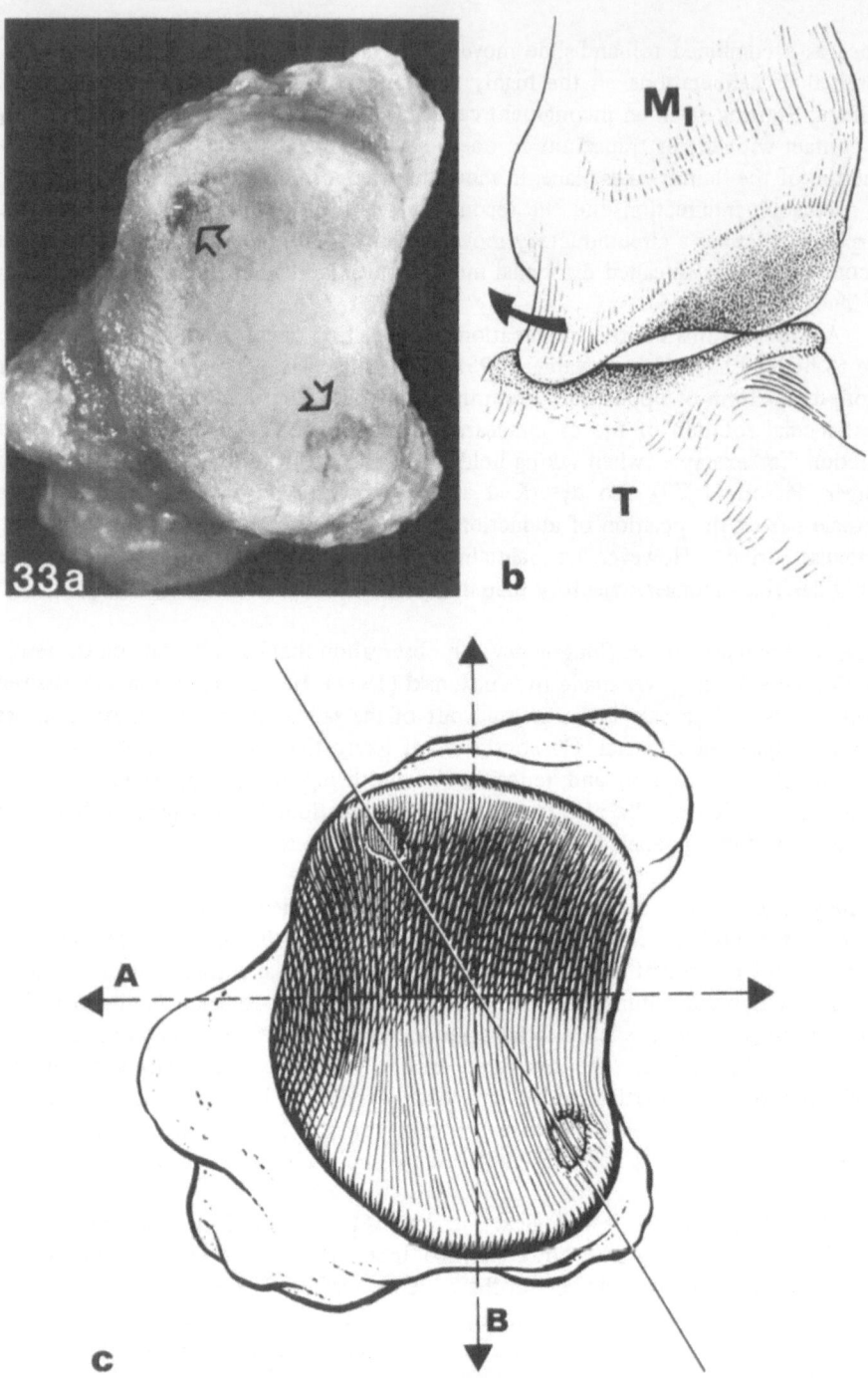

Fig. 33. Rotation in the thumb saddle joint: *a* The two cartilage lesions (*arrows*) on the os trapezium are diametrically opposite each other on the rising surface of the saddle arms. *b* During opposition, the metacarpal saddle can be seen to twist out of the os trapezium bed. *c* Projection of the abduction/adduction axis (*A*) and the flexion/extension axis (*B*) on the trapezial surface. The two lesions are joined by a line. The angle between this line and the flexion/extension axis (*b*) indicates the amount of rotation. (*a* and *b* after Koebke and Thomas 1979a)

The degree of rotation can be roughly determined by the cartilage lesions on the diametrically opposite os trapezium (Fig. 33c). To do this, the abduction/adduction axis and the flexion/extension axis are projected onto the trapezial surface. The chord connecting the dorsal and palmar tips of the saddle arm on the os metacarpale I (equal to the diameter of the dorsopalmar surface) lies along the flexion/extension axis when the joint is in the central position. The angle between the flexion/extension axis and a straight line connecting the cartilage lesions represents the degree of rotation of the metacarpus. The angle that could be measured by this method varied between $17°$ and $32°$. The considerable variation in values is due to the highly varied individual shape of the saddle joint, commented on also by Schmidt and Lieb (1981). According to their measurements, corresponding articular surfaces show no regularity in the distribution of their curvature profiles or in the diameter of the relevant curves. General statements of the value of maximal rotation, given by Henle (1855) as $40°$, by Du Bois-Reymond (1896) as $30°$, by De La Caffinière (1970) and by Dahhan et al. (1980) as about $15°$, do not take the different articular surfaces into consideration and, therefore, also neglect the individually varying degree of rotation of the thumb saddle joint.

Incongruence between joint surfaces is an important factor determining degenerative joint alteration (Preiser 1908; Pauwels 1976; Maquet 1976; Tillmann 1977; Brade and Koebke 1979). The fact that the articular surfaces "don't fit properly" leads to a reduction in the load-transferring contact area, which in turn results in a rise in compressive joint stress. If an upper limit of σ_0 (Tillmann 1978) is exceeded, cartilage lesions occur (Pauwels 1963, 1968).

Stress Distribution in a Model Test. The stress arising in the thumb saddle joint can be demonstrated in a model. When a model of the articulatio carpometacarpea pollicis with a congruent joint closure is subjected to load, stress distribution is equal in both joint members. There are no stress peaks in the sequence or relative height of the consecutive isochrome numbers in either half of the joint. However, if incongruency between the os trapezium and the os metacarpale I is simulated, stress peaks may be observed. The position and number of the isochromes show that the relative amount of joint pressure is extremely high around the small contact areas.

The results of photoelastic simulation tests permit the conclusion that the thumb saddle joint is subjected to uniform pressure under load in a congruent joint position. However, a particular mechanical stress arises during opposition when the metacarpus is medially rotated. This movement results in joint incongruency, whereby the small hollows in the articular cartilage that were occasionally observed must be seen as the direct morphological correlates of localized overloading of the cartilage. These cartilage lesions caused by mechanical stress may be considered the first stage in the development of arthrosis of the thumb saddle joint (Koebke and Thomas 1979a).

Tangential Fiber Layer of the Articular Cartilage as "Verkörpertes Spannungsfeld." The tangential fiber layer of the articular cartilage has been termed a *"verkörpertes Spannungsfeld"* (Pauwels 1959) — a physical field of tension. The collagen fiber bundles, resistent to tensile forces, are orientated trajectorially. They follow the line of the expansion trajectories in a model made of homogeneous material. The split lines, as already shown by Hultkranz (1898), reflect the organization of the collagen fiber bundles in the tangential fiber layer of the cartilage (Pauwels 1959; Konermann 1971;

Molzberger 1973; Tillmann 1978). Functional analysis of the split line pattern permits conclusions to be drawn about the stress to which a joint has been subjected, as it has been shown that strain has an effect on the organization of the collagen fibers.

The Interpretation of the Split Line Patterns. A uniform, basic split line pattern can be detected for the articular surface of the os metacarpale I. In the central part, the lines run parallel to each other through the dorsopalmar diameter of the oval articular surface. In the radial and ulnar parts of the saddle, they are increasingly deviated from straight lines by an attractive singular point on each side (Fig. 29a).

On the distal trapezial surface, two basic patterns occur with roughly equal frequency. Where the articular surface is square or rectangular in shape, there are four bow-shaped bundles of split lines that arise at the edges of the surface (cf. Fig. 29b) and avoid a repulsive singular point in the center. Where the articular surface is more triangular or rather S-shaped, there are three sets of curves (cf. Fig. 29c). An additional set of split lines occurring in two cases is a modification of the four-sided pattern.

Pauwels (1959) carried out photoelastic model tests and produced stress trajectories corresponding to the basic split line patterns. If an oval surface of homogeneous material (gelatine) is compressed so that pressure rises from the center towards the periphery, the course of the stress trajectories is identical to the split line pattern on the metacarpal articular surface.

If a rectangular slab is subjected to uniform pressure, the stress trajectories correspond to the split line pattern found on the os trapezium, where four bow-shaped sets of lines avoid a repulsive singular point. Uniform pressure on a triangular slab leads, as expected, to three sets of stress trajectories. When the course of the stress trajectories and the split line pattern are in such close correspondence, it can be considered unlikely, if not impossible, that this correspondence should be coincidental (Kummer 1959; Pauwels 1959; Konermann 1971). The course of the trajectories and of the split lines will only be the same if the pressure on the model corresponds to that on the articular surface.

This means that cartilage compression is roughly uniform over the surface of the os trapezium in the thumb saddle joint, while the cartilage of the articular surface of the os metacarpale I is subjected to more pressure at the edges than in the center. Increased peripheral compression of the radial and ulnar saddle arms of the os metacarpale I is the result of abduction and adduction in the thumb saddle joint. According to Du Bois-Reymond (1896), Bausenhardt (1949/50), Napier (1955), Kuczynski (1974), Schmidt and Lieb (1981), and our own findings (Koebke and Thomas 1979a), the radioulnar convex curvature of the os metacarpale I is greater than the corresponding concave curvature of the os trapezium. This means that abduction and adduction from a central position where the joint fissure is not closed will lead to a final position where the peripheral radial and ulnar surface areas are subjected to increasing compression.

Repulsive and Attractive Singular Points in the Split Line Pattern. The attractive and repulsive singular points found in the split line patterns are characteristic of each pattern (Pauwels 1959). Whereas a repulsive singular point may be regarded as a point of low stress, there is high compression surrounding an attractive singular point (Pauwels 1959; Konermann 1971; Molzberger 1973). Molzberger (1973) and Tillmann (1971, 1973, 1978) were able to show a correlation between the localization of attractive singular points and first occurrences of degenerative arthrotic cartilage deficiency. Cartilage lesions were found to occur close to attractive singular points both in the hip and elbow joint. This means that they occur in places where the joint stress is already high under normal conditions. This kind of clear relation cannot be established for the metacarpal articular surface of the thumb saddle joint on the basis of the present data. The cartilage lesions observed here were found in the palmar and dorsal saddle parts, while the attractive singular points were in the radial and ulnar regions.

If the results of split line analysis are summarized, we can state that the articular cartilage of the two joint members of the thumb saddle joint indicate functional adaptation to the "normal" movements occurring in a saddle joint. The articular cartilage is suited to abduction and adduction, flexion and extension, but not to rotation. Oppositional movement results in strain on the articulatio carpometacarpea pollicis like that on a ball-and-socket joint (Thomas 1977; Koebke and Thomas 1979a, b). The physiological rotation of the os metacarpale I leads to joint incongruence and stress peaks on the articular surfaces. This kind of particular functional strain of the thumb saddle joint explains early evidence of degenerative defects of the cartilage.

The Joint Capsule and Ligaments of the Thumb Saddle Joint. The unusual functional role of the articulatio carpometacarpea pollicis is partly due to the particular shape of the two joint members, but also to the capsule and ligaments which allow a wide range of movement. Henle (1855) and Hyrtl (1885) described the capsule as wide and loose. There is normally no contact between the joint cavity and neighboring joints (Henke 1863). It is an independent joint. There have, however, been rare cases documented arthrographically where there was a natural connection with the articulatio radiocarpea (H. Haage 1979, personal communication). The capsular wall is reinforced under the tendons of the long thumb muscles (Von Lanz and Wachsmuth 1959). Many studies have concentrated on the course of the intracapsular ligaments and their influence on the movements of the thumb saddle joint. Two reinforcing ligaments were described by R. Fick (1911), Poirier and Charpy (1911), and Eaton and Littler (1969). A palmar ligament runs diagonally from the tuberculum ossis trapezii in an ulnar direction to the tip of the base of the os metacarpale I. A similar, corresponding ligament runs on the dorsal side of the joint. In addition to these two diagonal ligaments, Haines (1944), Napier (1955), Kapandji (1963), De La Caffinière (1970), Pieron (1973), Bojsen-Møller (1976), Lewis (1977), and Dahhan et al. (1980) found a straight third ligament reinforcing the capsule on the radial side.

Although these ligaments described by the authors are strong, they don't reduce the laxity of the capsule. This was shown by Kuczynski (1974) on a prepared joint, where slight traction enabled him to separate the two articular surfaces by 3 mm. Adler (1975) examined normal stability of the thumb saddle joint of 50 healthy subjects and measured an average radial subluxation of 3.3 mm (maximum 7 mm). The relative instability of the thumb saddle joint is doubtless partly due to the positioning of the palmar and dorsal diagonal ligaments. A similar sitation was shown by Landsmeer (1955) to apply to the other fingers. The S-shaped positioning of the collateral ligaments of these fingers enables adduction of the extended finger to take place, and the articular surfaces may be distracted a little. On the other hand, it is the diagonal capsular ligaments that are usually accepted as the elements that make rotation in the joint possible during opposition of the thumb (Fick 1911; Haines 1944; Bausenhardt

1949/50; Brown 1970; Pieron 1973; Landsmeer 1976). The diagonal volar ligament causes supinate rotation during reposition, while the dorsal diagonal ligament leads to pronatal rotation of the os metacarpale I with increasing flexion (Bausenhardt 1949/50). In each case, the ligaments are taut in the final position, so that they hinder too much opposition or reposition (Von Lanz and Wachsmuth 1959). In opposition, they increase the incongruency of the joint closure resulting from the metacarpal saddle being turned and raised (Kuczynski 1974; Thomas 1977; Koebke and Thomas 1979a) and thus further increase the local stress at the articular surfaces. As described above, it is the local increase in stress due to rotation and incongruence that is assumed to be a causal factor leading to arthritic cartilage deficiencies.

Capsular Ligaments, Adductive Malposition, and Radial Subluxation. In advanced stages of thumb saddle joint arthrosis, clearly defective adduction has been observed in the thumb saddle joint (De Seze and Ryckewaert 1954; Aune 1955; Schlegel 1965; Pfiffner 1971; Helbig and Steinbach 1978). The malposition is caused by contraction of the musculi adductor pollicis and interosseus dorsalis primus, and is accompanied by (Bergk and Thümler 1979) or due to (Forestier 1937; Pfiffner 1971) radial subluxation of the os metacarpale I. Roentgenograms of this phenomenon (Pfiffner 1971; Thomas 1977; Segmüller 1978; Bergk and Thümler 1979) show palmar surface contact and a gapping joint cleft on the radial side. These clinical observations confirm macroscopic findings in dissected thumb saddle joints. The partial, palmar loss of cartilage on both articular surfaces is due to the unphysiological increase in joint pressure on the palmar surface caused by the defective adduction (Fig. 34a). In such cases of defective articular surfaces, a further small, localized defect is found, regularly at least on the trapezium (Fig. 34b), on the area that is still otherwise covered by a cartilage layer. This corresponds to one of the two small, diametrically opposed primary lesions typical of the early stages of rhizarthrosis. This result is another indication supporting the hypothesis that thumb saddle joint arthrosis begins with small, mechanically caused lesions and develops from there.

As already mentioned, the os metacarpale I shows an increasing tendency to subluxation in arthritic joints. Adler (1975) showed that, owing to the normal looseness of a healthy joint, individual dislocation can be excessive. Where there is also pathological weakness of the capsular ligaments, this is often seen as the cause of the arthrosis and the tendency for the metacarpus to dislocate (Aune 1955; Eaton and Littler 1969; Pfiffner 1971; Siegrist 1980). Mannerfeld (1978) observed a lesion of the volar diagonal ligament following bruising or spraining of the thumb ("a Bennett fracture without a fracture"). The ligament damage led to capsule weakness and to the secondary appearance of a posttraumatic form of arthrosis deformans. Mannerfeld (1978) suggested that degeneration of the volar diagonal ligament leads to idiopathic forms of thumb saddle joint arthrosis. Swanson (1980) noted that it was usually necessary to replace the "often insufficient ventral diagonal ligament" when operating for rhizarthrosis. At the same time, the base of the os metacarpale I should be attached to that of the os metacarpale II.

The Ligamentum Metacarpeum Dorsale I. This kind of connection between the first and second metacarpal bones is found in healthy joints in the form of a ligament between the two bones, documented by dissection of the joints. This ligamentum metacarpeum dorsale I typically arises from a dorsoradial spur at the base of the second

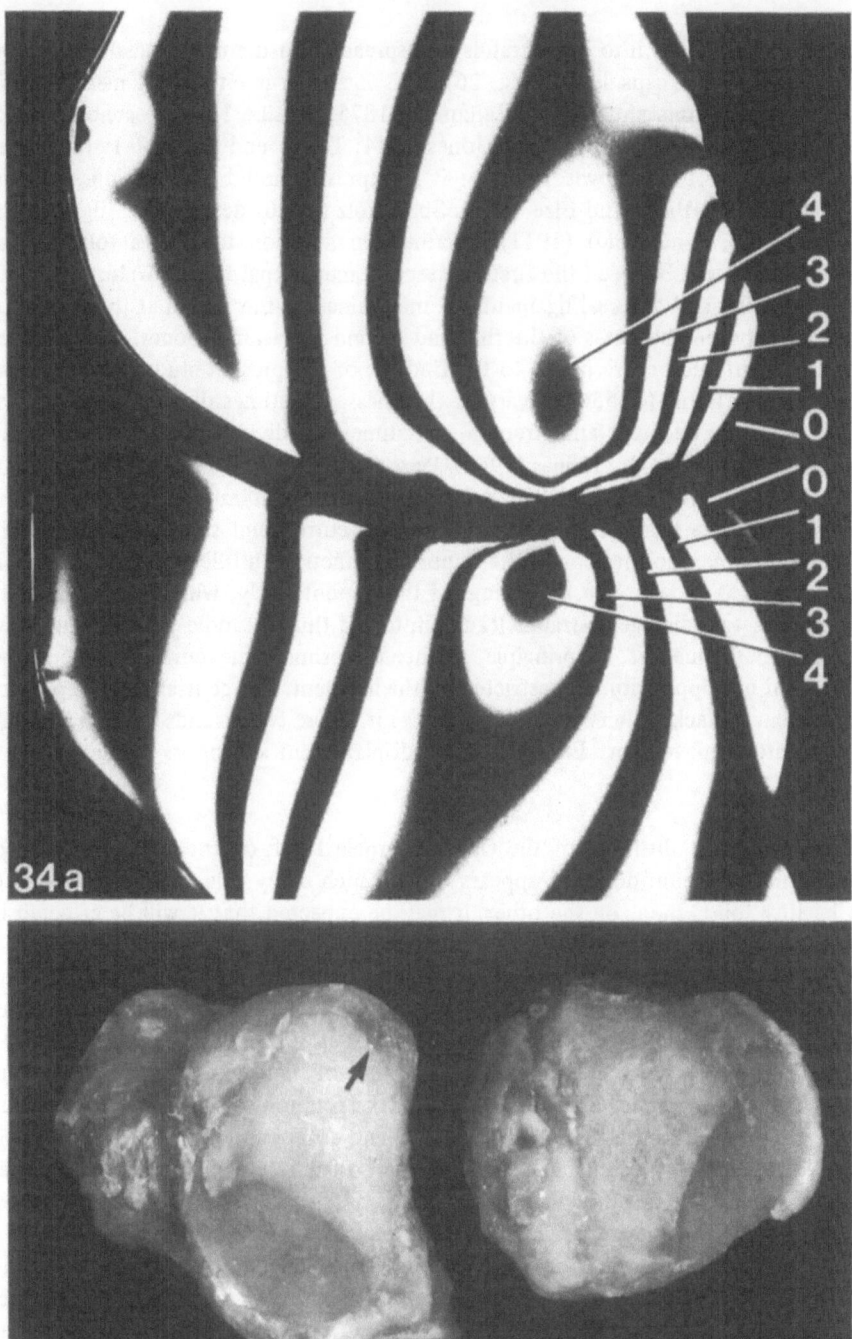

Fig. 34. *a* Photoelastic experiment to show excentric load. Compressive stress is greater on the right than on the left. The isochrome with the highest ordinal number, 4, has slipped to the right. The experiment simulates pressure in the thumb saddle joint during malpositioned adduction of the os metacarpale I. Joint pressure is pathologically high in the palmar zone. *b* Left saddle joint of a 57-year-old man. The articular surfaces of the first metacarpal bone (*right*) and the os trapezium (*left*) are free of cartilage in the palmar regions. The trapezial surface shows a further small defect (*arrow*) typical for early stages of rhizarthrosis

metacarpus. It divides into two strands and spreads into the ulnar-radial part of the thumb saddle joint capsule (cf. Fig. 26). This ligament is either not mentioned in anatomic descriptions and atlases (Heitzmann 1875; Brösike 1892; Gegenbaur 1895; von Langer and Toldt 1911; Wood Jones 1944; Testut and Latarjet 1948; Napier 1955, Sieglbauer 1958; Lewis 1977) or it is expressly noted as being missing (von Bardeleben 1906; Braus and Elze 1954). Spalteholz (1896) described a "ligamentum basium dorsale," and Toldt (1911) described, in addition to this, a volar and an interosseal ligament between the first and second metacarpal bones. Waldeyer (1950) depicted a volar and a dorsal ligament but maintained in the text that there were no ligaments between the bases of the first and second metacarpal bones. A description of the ligaments that corresponds to the findings of the present study may be found in the work of Henle (1855: "of varying thickness, sometimes divided") and R. Fick (1911: "varies in its shape and strength, sometimes it is divided in two strands"). The ligament was also noted by Haines (1944), Pieron (1973), and De La Caffinière (1970). Bojsen-Møller (1976) referred more clearly to its functional importance. Although his description of the ligament positioning does not correspond to the findings of the present study, he also mentioned the important function fulfilled by the ligament in fastening the os metacarpale I. Findings of the present study, which suggest that the ligament has two divergent strands leading into the thumb saddle joint capsule, have functional consequences. In principle, neither the primary movements of the thumb saddle joint nor opposition are restricted by the ligament. In a central, neutral position the ligament is slack, otherwise one strand is taut. These two strands serve to passively guide rotatory movement. Extreme radial displacement of the os metacarpale I is prevented.

The Bone Spur at the Base of the Os Metacarpale II. If, on the one hand, the ligamentum metacarpeum dorsale I appears to play such a key role in the functioning of the healthy joint, then, on the other, it may be expected that it will be affected by degenerative processes involving the arthritic joint.

A bone spur, evident at the base of the os metacarpale II in seven hands from corpses, gives morphological evidence of a degenerative change in the ligamentum metacarpeum dorsale I (cf. Fig. 25c). Thomas et al. (in press) evaluated 1493 roentgenograms of the hand and found this kind of bone spur in 116 cases. As has been shown, this spur corresponds to the point of fixation of the ligament at the base of the second metacarpal bone (cf. Fig. 27). The development of an exostotic bone spur at the point of attachment of a ligament is most simply explained by tensile stress occurring there. In its function as a restrictor for the os metacarpale I, one or both strands of the ligament are pulled taut. The point at the base of the os metacarpale II is the punctum fixum when the ligament is under tensile load, while the two strands running into the joint capsule are free to move. According to Pauwels (1960), ossification of the ligament is only to be expected at the point of fixation on the second metacarpus. In keeping with the theory of causal histogenesis, bone tissue can develop without any particular stress being exerted, provided there is a fairly static tissue frame in the form of connective tissue, cartilage, or bone (Pauwels 1960). Koebke and Tillmann (1977) were able to show the process of ossification in the case of the temporal styloid process as an example of a rigid tissue subjected to constant tensile stress. Ligament ossification is due, according to Weidenreich (1923), to "constant even strain" or "overloading." Schneider H (1959), Schneider PG (1964), and Becker and

Krahl (1978) believed the cause for bone spur development to lie purely in mechanical stimulus in the form of overloading.

The bone structure in the immediate vicinity of the ligament attachment point shows, in individual cases, clear spongiosa in the traction direction of the ligament. This clearly shows the functional adaptation of the bone itself to the stress brought about by the ligament. The computer-aided quantitative evaluation of roentgenograms shows thickening of the ligament close to the os metacarpale II (see Fig. 30), corresponding to granular calcium deposits in the histologically prepared and examined material (cf. Fig. 31). The development of calcium salt crystals either leads to final fibroostotic ligament alteration, or the bone spur is provided with appositional growth.

If, on the one hand, the development of the bone spur can be seen as an indication of tensile load on the ligament, on the other hand, degenerative stretching of the ligament may be expected to occur with time. The lack of elasticity of the ligament caused by stretching means that the os metacarpale I loses a functionally important guiding and retaining support. In particular, if the ligament becomes stretched, then pathological subluxation of the first metacarpus must be expected. This again leads to the defective positioning typical of many cases of thumb saddle joint arthrosis.

The analysis of clinical roentgenograms indicates with a high degree of probability (Thomas et al., in press) that a bone spur will occur concomitant with arthrosis. This type of connection is documented in serial roentgenograms (Thomas et al., in press).

3.5 Conclusions

If available results and their interpretations are summarized, it would appear that the genesis of rhizarthrosis takes place in four stages.
1. The essentially physiological rotational movement in the thumb saddle joint leads to loss of articular surface contact and thus to joint incongruence with localized stress peaks. Minor lesions of the articular cartilage on the side parts of the saddle are mechanically caused, early signs of arthritic change.
2. The contractive adduction defect in the thumb saddle joint causes compressive joint forces in the palmar region of the articular surfaces that are far greater than normal physiological strain. The cartilage degenerates and partial arthritic "bald spots" appear.
3. The ligamentum metacarpeum dorsale I is already stretched or becomes so, losing its elasticity and its function as a retainer for the os metacarpale I. The radial subluxation tendency of the first metacarpus increases. Degenerative joint alteration affects the radial part of the articular surfaces.
4. Advanced arthrosis of the thumb saddle joint is characterized by severe deformation of the two joint members. Osteophytes are usually found both on the os metacarpale I and on the os trapezium. Fixed subluxation of the os metacarpale I is frequently observed (Forestier 1937; Müller 1949; De Seze and Ryckewaert 1954; Bergk and Thümler 1979), which is assisted by radial sloping of the trapezial surface. There are often free-floating bodies in the joint where thumb saddle joint arthrosis occurs (Geschwend 1970; Koebke and Thomas 1979a).

These unattached particles are to be expected in various types of joint disease, according to Klein and Huth (1980). They are due to correspondingly different causes. In the case of rhizarthrosis, however, it appears probable that they originate from exostoses that break off (Horvath and Lengyel 1976). This hypothesis is supported by their position at the edge of the joint capsule and their connection to it. The possibility cannot be excluded that a secondary arthrosis deformans might be caused by one of these bodies being trapped between surfaces (Klein and Huth 1980).

The articulatio carpometacarpea pollicis of the human hand, as a joint with saddle-shaped articular surfaces, is functionally adapted to abduction/adduction and to flexion/extension. However, if it is subjected to strain as if it were a ball-and-socket joint, this leads to particular mechanical stress. Physiological rotation in connection with opposition of the thumb — facilitated by the capsule itself and the ligaments — leads to loss of joint congruency. Results of the present study support the hypothesis that the causes of arthrosis are rooted in this increase in mechanical stress due to incongruency. These findings complement clinical observations that people whose work involves coordinated thumb movement including opposition frequently suffer from arthrosis of the thumb saddle joint (Cotta and Mittelmeier 1959; Thomas 1977).

Replacement of the thumb saddle joint in extreme cases of joint deficiency by an endoprothesis functionally corresponding to a ball-and-socket joint is in keeping with the normal physiological function of the joint (Thomas 1977).

Comparative anatomic studies with primates have shown that the articulatio carpometacarpea pollicis is normally a ball-and-socket joint in *Hylobates* (Napier and Napier 1967) and sometimes also in *Pongo pygmaeus* (Lewis 1977).

4 Metacarpophalangeal Joints

4.1 Introduction

Almost all actions carried out with the hand rely on proper functioning of the metacarpophalangeal joints. They are used in the various kinds of grip requiring strength and also for modification of fingertip or precision action. The individual function of each finger in actions performed by the hand requires special positioning of the metacarpophalangeal joints and causes a given strain on the joints. According to Brown (1970) and Hazelton et al. (1975), it is the middle finger, ring finger, and little finger that provide the necessary strength for a firm grip. The metacarpophalangeal joints are bent. The index finger and thumb function as retainers, making the grip more precise without being under so much load themselves. Their metacarpophalangeal joints are then usually extended. Stability in the fingertip hold is usually achieved by the index finger with a bent metacarpophalangeal joint and by the thumb with the joint extended (Chao et al. 1976).

From a morphological point of view, the articulationes metacarpophalangeae II–V are ball-and-socket joints. The biconcavely indented end of the metacarpal bone articulates with the smaller phalangeal socket. Joint stability is mainly provided for by the side ligaments (Segmüller 1978) and the palmar fibrous cartilage disk. The sturdy ligamentum palmare, in which there is often a sesamoid bone at the base of the index finger and the little finger (Pfitzner 1892, Joseph 1951b), functions as a guide for the long flexor tendons. During movement in the joint, it glides around the radioulnar axis on to the palmar-facing surface of the side parts of the joints of the ossa metacarpalia II–V.

Functionally, the metacarpophalangeal joint of the four fingers is restricted to active movement around two axes. However, in addition to flexion/extension and abduction/adduction, rotary movement does occur in connection with these main actions (Fick 1904, 1911; Landsmeer 1955; Landsmeer and Ansingh 1957; Brown 1970; Lewis 1977). The extent and direction of rotary movement varies from finger to finger. Rotation occurs as a function of closing the hand to form a fist, and also is a prerequisite for hollowing the palm and rounding the back of the hand (Braune 1887; Krmpotić-Nemanić 1967; Flatt 1974).

In his description of the thumb, R. Fick (1911) stated that "to a certain extent the thumb loses in freedom of movement what it has gained in the saddle joint, i.e., in the carpometacarpal joint." Other researchers (e.g., Swanson 1972; Hirsch et al. 1974) are also of the opinion that the metacarpophalangeal joint of the thumb is both morphologically and functionally a hinge joint. Whereas Von Lanz and Wachsmuth (1959) described this joint, like the interphalangeal joints, as having a hollow in the top of the os metacarpale I and ridged articular socket at the base of the lowest phalanx, this view is refuted by Reimann and Ebner (1980).

Referring to the metacarpophalangeal thumb joint as a ginglymus is often based on the hypothesis that the thumb originally had three joints. It has been postulated that the os metacarpale I contributed to the formation of the os trapezium and that the metacarpus of the two-jointed thumb is really the lowest phalanx (Hyrtl 1885; Gräfenberg 1914; Siegert 1930; Faller 1980). The position of the growth plate and the foramen nutricium are thereby considered to be morphological phenomena that support this hypothesis. However, like other hypotheses, this may be considered too speculative and unfounded (Müller 1937; Ferber 1953; Koebke 1980), and does not justify a classification of this joint as one of the interphalangeal joints.

The morphological variation in the metacarpal head (Harris and Joseph 1949; Joseph 1951a) determines the individual freedom of flexion of the metacarpophalangeal thumb joint (Parsons 1895; Joseph 1951a). However, according to Reimann and Ebner (1980), this variation has no effect on the degree of active movement possible to the side in an ulnar direction, as shown by their findings. Du Bois-Reymond (1896) maintained that active rotation in the metacarpophalangeal thumb joint was 30° during opposition.

In the following section of this study, the exterior form of the joint members of the metacarpophalangeal joints and the spongiosa architecture close to the joint ends of the relevant bones are examined. Findings are discussed in the light of the functional strain on these joints. In addition, an attempt is made to relate typical morphological characteristics of the individual joint to the specific strain placed on each finger when the hand is used. To this end, the results of photoelastic experiments are correlated with the analysis of spongiosa architecture and of the split line pattern on the articular cartilage.

4.2 Material and Methods

The articulationes metacarpophalangeae II–V were examined from the hands of 14 adults (aged 30 to 76) and six children (aged 3 to 4).

The metacarpophalangeal joint of the thumb was examined on the same hands as had been used to analyze the thumb saddle joint (from 21 adult males and 13 adult females, aged 25 to 96). Roentgenograms were prepared of these 68 joints (see Sect. 3.2).

4.2.1 Macroscopic Examination and Split Line Production and Documentation

The joints were largely free of soft tissue and were opened up for macroscopic examination by severing one of the two collateral ligaments, in order to avoid damage to the articular surfaces. Cartilage alterations on the metacarpal and phalangeal articular surfaces were sketched or photographed.

Split lines were produced on the proximal and distal articular surfaces of the metacarpophalangeal joints II–V of 14 adult and 3 child hands. The split line pattern of the first metacarpophalangeal joint was examined in 20 cases (method according to Konermann, see Sect. 2.2.2). In order to interpret the split lines, the pattern on the convex articular surface of the ossa metacarpalia must be represented on a flat surface. To do this, the bone was fastened to a stand that could be rotated. The bone was turned 40°–50° between each photograph. The scale remained constant. This permitted the split line pattern to be fully documented in three or four photographs. Photos were enlarged 8–10 times and put together for each joint surface. Overlapping of the photos meant that distortion was not very great. The metacarpal thumb joint surface is less convex, so that two photos were usually sufficient to represent the entire split line pattern.

4.2.2 Photoelastic Experiments

Models were made of the distal and proximal articular surfaces of the second to fifth metacarpophalangeal joints and were analyzed in order to see how far the split line pattern corresponded to stress trajectories induced experimentally by pressure application. To do this, 0.7–1 cm thick layers of aspic were poured onto a flat glass surface. When the aspic had set, the models were subjected to pressure by placing another glass sheet on top in apparatus modified on the basis of Molzberger (1973). Like other homogeneous transparent material, aspic shows double refraction under pressure. If the model under pressure is placed between the analyzer and the polarizer of the photoelastic apparatus, isoclines appear in the model in linearly polarized light. Isoclines are lines in which the stress trajectories run in the same direction. Establishing and indicating stress trajectories on the basis of isoclines was done according to Kummer's (1959) photographic method. Detailed theoretical issues concerning the photoelastic measuring method were discussed by Föppl and Mönch (1950) and by Kummer (1959). Pauwels (1959) showed that the results obtained from a homogeneous model can be related to those to be expected from articular cartilage.

To produce and analyze the stress trajectories on the dorsopalmar surface of the distal metacarpal joint member, two-dimensional models were made using 10-mm-thick Plexiglas.

4.2.3 Roentgenograms, Equidensity Measurements, and Histological Examination

In order to analyze the spongiosa architecture and to determine the distribution of material in the bone, 2-mm-thick planar midsagittal sections were cut from the ossa metacarpalia I–V and roentgenograms were made of the respective phalanges (Definix Medical Kodak, 100 mAS, 42 kV). An aluminum rule was included in the pictures to facilitate calibration (Bergerhoff 1944).

When the right X-ray film is used, not only the hard bone but also the articular cartilage is visible. This kind of roentgenogram is suitable for quantitative density analysis of the bone by computerized film analysis (Schleicher et al. 1980; see Sect. 3.2.1). The measurement printouts enable bone density to be related to cartilage thickness; absolute cartilage thickness was not measured.

Twelve metacarpal joint members were decalcified in EDTA solution and prepared for histological examination. Seventeen ulnar and 17 radial collateral ligaments from metacarpophalangeal joints II–V were histologically analyzed, together with 13 radial or ulnar capsule portions from joints II or V. Sections were cut through the ring finger and little finger at joint level from the hands of two newborns and one 4-year-old child.

4.3 Results

4.3.1 Macroscopic Findings and Results of Split Line Examination

The articular surface of the second to fifth metacarpal joint parts has two palmar extensions. In the case of the ossa metacarpalia III and IV, they are almost symmetrical in size and shape. On the index finger, the radial condylus is larger; on the little finger this applies to the ulnar condylus. The distal and palmar cartilage areas extend over the rounded edge of the articular surface to the ulnar and radial edges of the bone end. In the palmar region, this bow-shaped double cartilage strip is broader near the condylus than on the distal side (Fig. 35).

On the 14 hands examined, 8 were found to show macroscopically visible cartilage deficiencies on the articular surface of the metacarpophalangeal joints II—V. In five of these eight cases, lesions were found on more than one of the four joints. On the metacarpal side of the joint, the lesions occurred as localized spots or stripes in the palmar region of the articular surface (Fig. 36).

In a few cases, the lesions extended into the center of the articular surface. In one case, cartilage defects were only located in one clearly defined area on the ulnar surface of the third metacarpus. In two further cases, the index finger was characterized by a cartilage-free sulcus at the base of the radial condylus. In both of these cases, there was also a sesamoid bone in the ligamentum palmare (Fig. 37).

Degenerative cartilage alteration was found in the peripheral dorsal area of the oval articular socket of the first phalanx (Fig. 38a). In some cases, these lesions extended into the center of the concave area. Macroscopic examination of the 62 thumb joints that were opened showed 24 cases of pathological joint alteration in

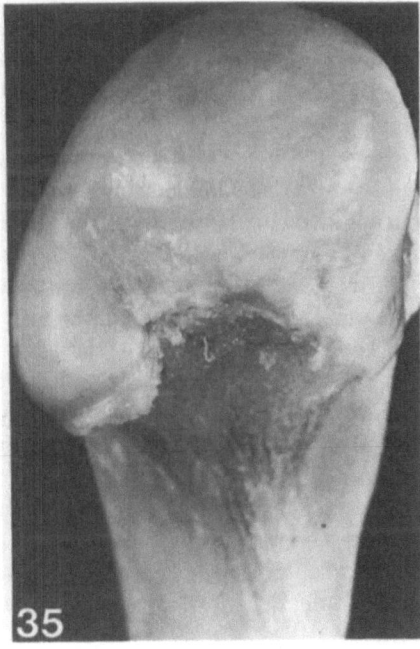

35

Fig. 35. Palmar view of the head of the left os metacarpale II (43-year-old woman) with asymmetric palmar condyles

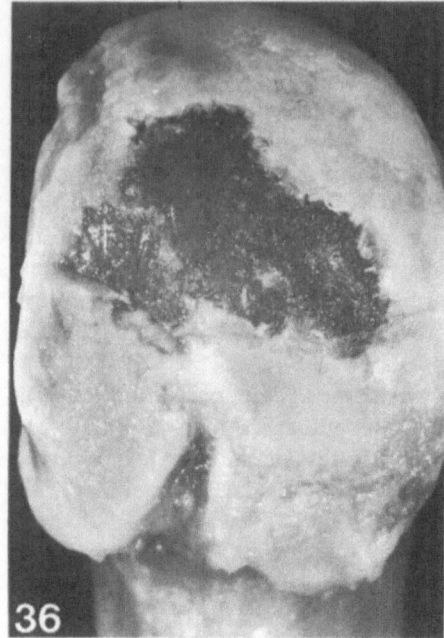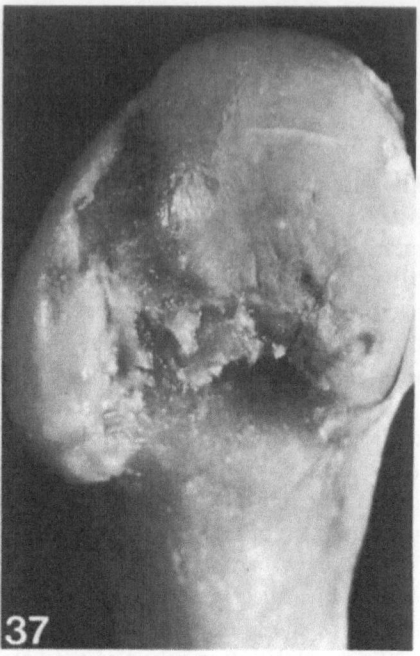

Fig. 36. Palmar-distal view of the right caput ossis metacarpalis V of a 79-year-old man. The cartilage has been destroyed in the palmar zone; the subchondral bone is exposed

Fig. 37. Palmar view of the left head of the os metacarpale II of an 80-year-old woman. The radial condylus is separated from the remaining surface area by a cartilage-free sulcus

varying degrees of severity. Where cartilage lesions occurred, these were almost always found on the radiopalmar part of the articular surface or across the entire radial area (Fig. 38b). In 17 cases, degeneration of the metacarpophalangeal joint was found to occur along with degeneration of the thumb saddle joint.

The Proximal Articular Surface. The split line pattern varied considerably on the ends of the ossa metacarpalia II–V. More than one third of the patterns found deviated from normal. The normal pattern is characterized by numerous parallel lines running across the long, dorsopalmar axis of the articular surface. There are two attractive singular points on both the radial side and the ulnar side. Between them, there is a repulsive singular point (Fig. 39). Modifications of the basic pattern affect both the central parallel lines and the attractive singular points at the sides. The parallel lines were found, for example, in some cases to remain parallel dorsally but to diverge on the palmar side or to take a radial turn (Fig. 40). The number of attractive singular points was found to be reduced by as much as three.

The split line pattern established for the head of the os metacarpale I was found to correspond basically to the normal pattern. The parallel split lines in the center of the articular surface were orientated towards the small dorsopalmar section. In four cases, the pattern was modified, and an additional ulnar curve was described by the lines.

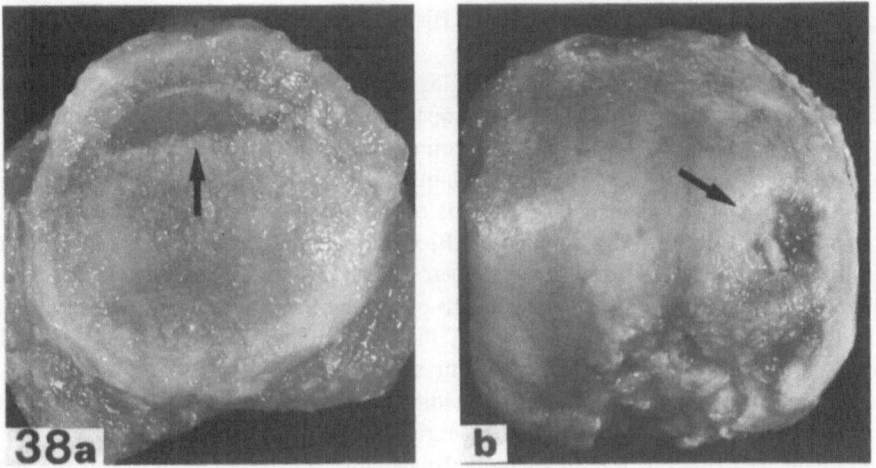

Fig. 38. *a* Top view of the joint socket of the phalanx proximalis of the left index finger of a 66-year-old man. A crescent-shaped cartilage lesion may be seen in the peripheral dorsal zone of the articular surface (→). *b* Distal view of the head of the right os metacarpale I (78-year-old man). On the radial side, a localized defect of the articular cartilage (→)

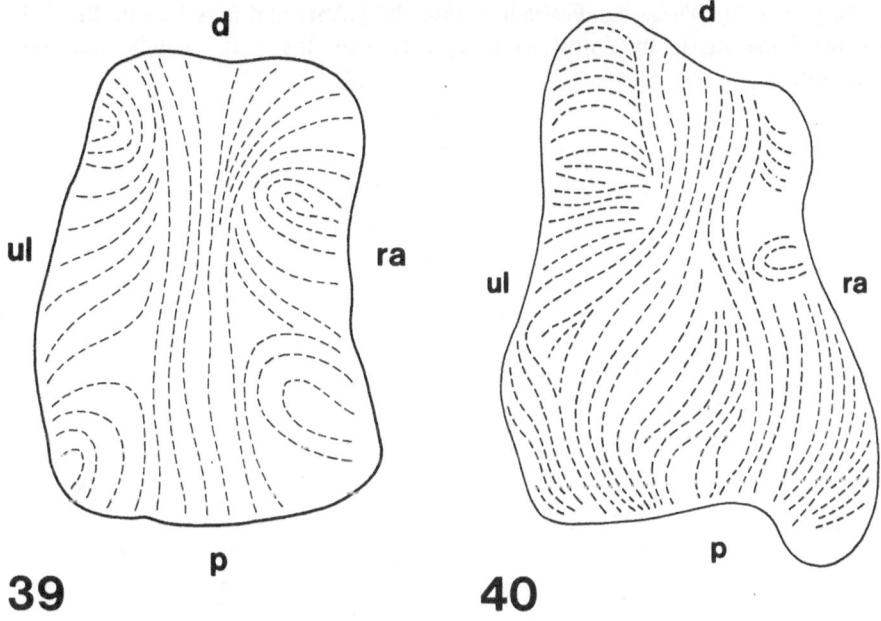

Fig. 39. Basic split line pattern on the metacarpal articular surface (*d*, dorsal; *p*, palmar; *ul*, ulnar; *ra*, radial)

Fig. 40. Split line pattern variant for the metacarpal articular surface

The Distal Articular Surface. The split lines on the oval concave joint surfaces of the first phalanges I–V were uniform in pattern. The most frequently observed pattern was made up of three bow-shaped sets of lines arising from the periphery and coming back to back around a central repulsive singular point (Fig. 41). In a few cases, the dorsal attractive singular point was missing.

4.3.2 Roentgenographic, Equidensity, and Histological Findings

Roentgenograms of 2-mm-thick planar midsagittal sections of ossa metacarpalia permitted the bone architecture in the dorsopalmar area to be studied. The caput ossis metacarpalis is filled with spongiosa. In young adults, spongiosa bundles may be seen running from the subchondral compact lamella at right angles, toward the center of the caput ossis metacarpalis II–V. There is an area of greater density that runs dorsopalmarly and is distally slightly concave. From this dense line, a dorsal and a palmar bundle of spongiosa can be discerned. These spongiosa bundles run toward the metaphysis into the dorsal and palmar corticalis of the bone shaft. They are medially limited by the marrow zone. In older adults, the dorsopalmar area of greater density is not visible or only weakly perceptible. The spongiosa that run from the subchondral lamella merge gradually with the two columns of spongiosa running into the shaft. Of these two, the dorsal one is sometimes rarified or absent (Fig. 42a).

In the head of the thumb os metacarpale, the spongiosa radiates from the subchondral lamella in two bundles straight into the palmar and dorsal metaphyseal corticalis. In many cases, the dorsal spongiosa reinforcement was clearly thin.

In the phalangeal bone ends of the same joints, I–V, spongiosa was found to run in two compact bundles in the dorsopalmar region, starting from the subchondral lamella (Fig. 42b). These bundles radiate into the palmar and dorsal corticalis of the proximal bone shaft. In almost all cases examined, the dorsal bundle was more prominent.

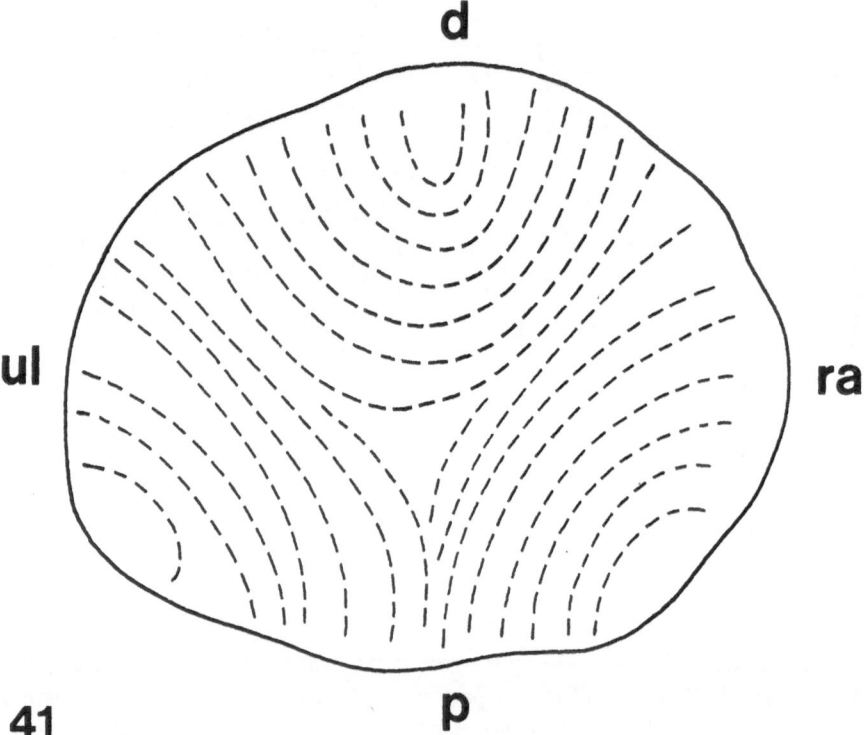

Fig. 41. Basic split line pattern on the phalangeal articular surface of the metacarpophalangeal joints

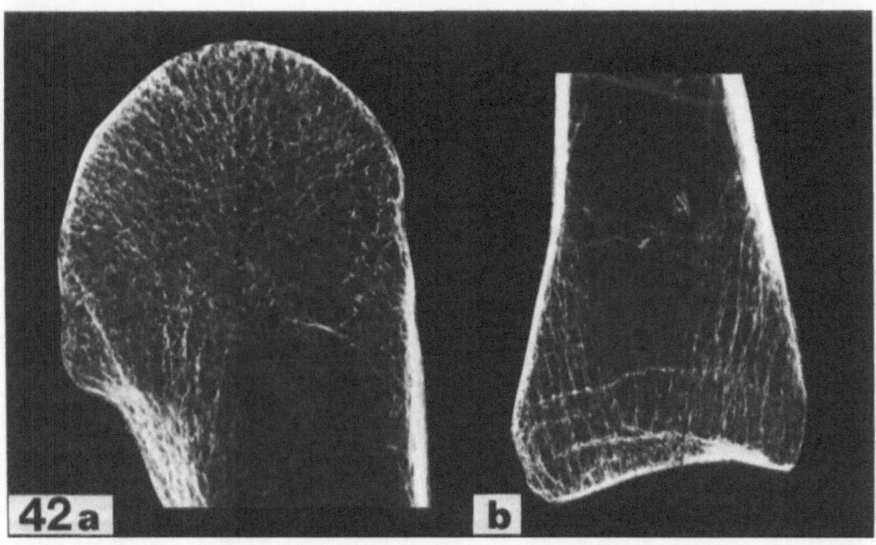

Fig. 42. *a* Roentgenogram of a 2-mm-thick midsagittal section through the head of the right os metacarpale III of a 73-year-old man. *b* Roentgenogram of a 2-mm-thick midsagittal section through the base of the corresponding first phalangeal bone

Equidenses of 2-mm-thick midsagittal sections of the distal part of the ossa metacarpalia II–V show the area of greatest bone density as a black area, corresponding to an aluminum probe thickness of $\geq$ 1 mm. These areas were found to lie in the palmar and dorsal corticalis in the metaphysis, and in the bone lamella under the cartilage of the bone head (Fig. 43). The subchondral compacta was found to decrease in thickness from the index finger successively to the little finger.

The articular cartilage corresponded to a 0.4 to 0.5-mm-thick aluminum probe in its X-ray absorption. On the os metacarpale II, the cartilage layer was found to be of uniform thickness in the palmar and central areas and to·be a little thinner dorsally. On the middle and ring fingers, the area where the cartilage was thickest was palmar, and this tendency was strongest on the little finger.

Examination of cross-sectional and frontal sections of metacarpal bone heads by light microscopy showed that the radial and ulnar side curved sections consisted of hyaline cartilage (Fig. 44a). Similarly, the radial and ulnar condyli on the· ossa metacarpalia II–V were covered with hyaline cartilage. In over half the cases examined, the ligamenta collateralia, consisting of layers of dense collagen fibers, contained groups of cartilage cells. These cells were found to lie in the inner part of the ligament, on the side closest to the joint cavity. Cartilage cells were also frequently found in the thickened, compact parts of the capsule opposite the radial condylus of the caput ossis metacarpalis II and the ulnar condylus of the little finger (Fig. 44b).

4.4 Discussion

The Morphology and Mechanics of the Metacarpophalangeal Joints II–V. The articulationes metacarpophalangeae II–V are morphologically ball-and-socket joints

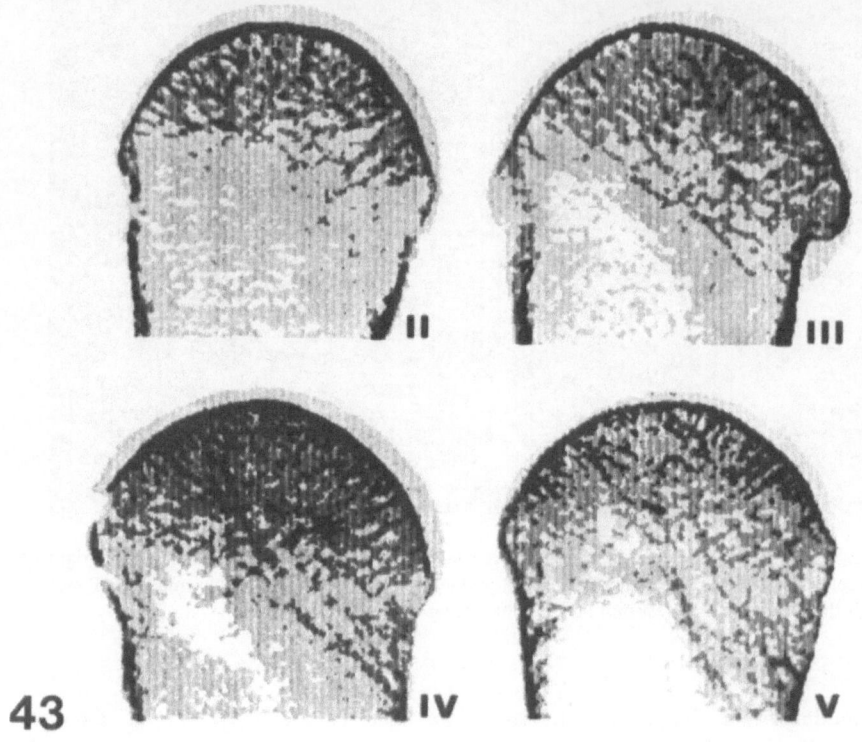

Fig. 43. Equidenses of 2-mm-thick midsagittal sections through the distal part of the ossa metacarpalia II–V (59-year-old man, left hand). Shades of gray correspond to aluminum absorption, given in mm

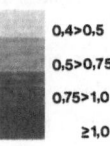

	0,4>0,5
	0,5>0,75
	0,75>1,0
	≥1,0

where, from a central position, dorsal extension and palmar flexion take place around a transverse axis. Abduction and adduction movements around a dorsopalmar axis are possible when the joint is extended or slightly bent. Rotation of the fingers occurs in conjunction with these main movements (Henle 1855; Fischer 1907), e.g., in connection with spreading the fingers. This phenomenon was explained by R. Fick (1904, 1911) and Landsmeer (1955) by the asymmetric positioning and differences in strength of the collateral ligaments. Contrary to the description offered in standard anatomical textbooks, the collateral ligaments of the metacarpophalangeal joints II–V are taut in every joint position (Landsmeer 1955), and lie close to the caput ossis metacarpalis.

This statement is supported by the development of ridges of hyaline cartilage at the radial and ulnar edges of the metacarpal heads. The taut ligaments lead to exertion of pressure at the sides, where these ridges are situated. If a ligament itself or a tendon is locally subjected to pressure rather than tension, cartilage cells are differentiated in the tissue around (Krompecher 1937; Ploetz 1938; Pauwels 1960; Altmann 1964; Tillmann and Konermann 1979).

The inner zone of the collateral ligaments, closest to the cartilage ridges, was found to contain numerous cartilage cells. These were not present in the outer parts

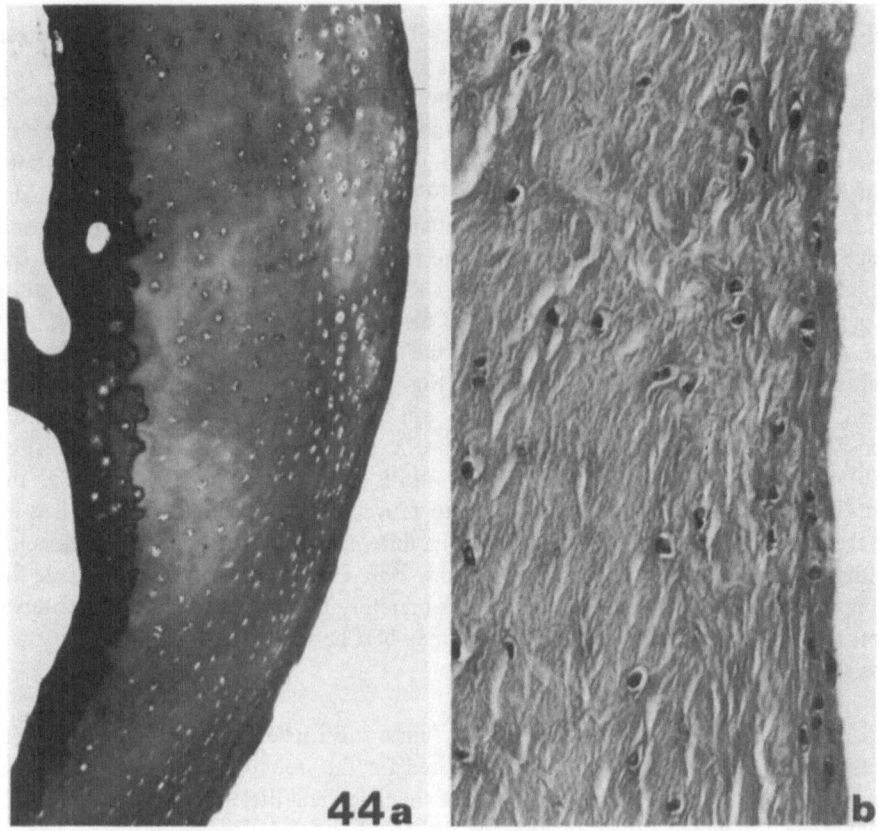

Fig. 44. *a* Histological section through the radial crest of the metacarpal head (left os metacarpale II, 71-year-old man) showing hyaline cartilage. Azan, 12 μm; × 42. *b* Histological section through the thickened radial capsule of the corresponding metacarpophalangeal joint. Goldner, 8 μm; × 75

of the ligaments. To correspond to the dominant tension stress occurring here, tissue structure mainly contains fibrocytes.

The collateral ligaments of the metacarpophalangeal joints II–V are not proximo-distally straight when the fingers are extended, but run diagonally in a distal-palmar direction (Henke 1863; Fick 1904; Landsmeer 1955). According to Landsmeer (1955), abduction/adduction of the extended finger is possible in spite of the taut collateral ligaments because these ligaments are straightened during this movement. This leads to rotation in combination with abduction/adduction (Landsmeer 1955; Landsmeer and Ansingh 1957).

The Asymmetrical Joint Surfaces of the Ossa Metacarpalia II and V. R. Fick (1904), Shiino (1925), Landsmeer (1955), and Lewis (1977) referred to the asymmetric shape of the palmar, condylic protuberances on the heads of the ossa metacarpalia II and V. Shiino (1925) and Lewis (1977) considered this compact, rounded radial or ulnar protuberance on the index finger and little finger to cause rotation of the finger in conjunction with flexing movements and increasing tension of the relevant collateral ligament. When it is bent, the index finger rotates inwardly towards the middle finger (pronation), while the little finger describes a movement of supination (Lewis 1977). Contrary to the opinion expressed by Shiino (1925), there is no contact between the oval articular surface of the first phalanx and the radial or ulnar condylus during this movement. Even when the finger is bent at right angles, roentgenography demonstrates that the phalangeal articular surface is clearly separate from the relevant protuberance.

A functional explanation for the existence of these cartilage-covered radial and ulnar protuberances on the index finger and little finger is offered by analysis of the topographic relations between skeletal parts and muscles in the region of these joints (Koebke and Stümpel 1981). Cross-sections through the index finger show clearly that the m. interosseus dorsalis primus and the first lumbrical muscle pass over the condylus on the radial side of the joint (Fig. 45a). The joint capsule lying between them is thickened at this point and inlaid with cartilage cells. On the little finger, the mm. abductor and flexor digiti minimi brevis run across the ulnar condylus (Fig. 45b). On both fingers, the protuberance fulfills the function of a fulcrum for the muscles. The ability of the index finger to move into a position of abduction is increased by the action of the first dorsal m. interosseus — which electromyographic findings (Tamega et al. 1980) indicate to have only an abduction function — while the same is true for the little finger of the m. abductor. This corresponds to the observation that the index finger and little finger may best be spread from the neutral central position (Fig. 45c).

Sesamoid Bones at the Basal Joint of the Index and Little Fingers. Under this functional aspect, a possible explanation is offered for the frequent occurrence of a radial or ulnar sesamoid bone at the basal joint of the index and little finger. Pfitzner (1892) established frequency values of 44% for the occurrence of a sesamoid bone adjacent to the index finger joint and 75% for the same phenomenon on the little finger; the findings of the present study support these values. On the index finger, the sesamoid bone in the palmar fibrous cartilage disk forms a volar and a radial platform for the m. lumbricalis primus. This acts on the radial side of the first phalanx, partly covering the volar part of the sesamoid bone (Fig. 46a). The supporting abductory action of the m. lumbricalis primus, as postulated by Braithwaite et al. (1948) and Von Lanz and Wachsmuth (1959) and affirmed by electromyographic examination (Backhouse and Catton 1954), seems to be particularly relevant where there is a sesamoid bone. An analogous mechanism for the m. flexor digiti minimi brevis on the little finger appears probable.

The view expressed by Henle (1855), that the sesamoid bone of the index finger and little finger glides on the relevant condylus during movement of the joint, cannot be supported. The degenerative, cartilage-free sulcus found on the articular surface of the second metacarpal bone in two cases was a clear indication of the path of the sesamoid bone between the protuberance and the actual articular surface. The one case observed by R. Fick (1904), where the condylus was "normally" separated from the main surface area, must be attributed to cartilage degeneration.

Spongiosa Architecture as a Trajectorial System. With the proper methods, morphological features can be analyzed and interpreted to show the physiological strain on a joint. The spongiosa structure in the dorsopalmar region of the two bones connected by the metacarpophalangeal joint gives evidence of compressive strain. Roent-

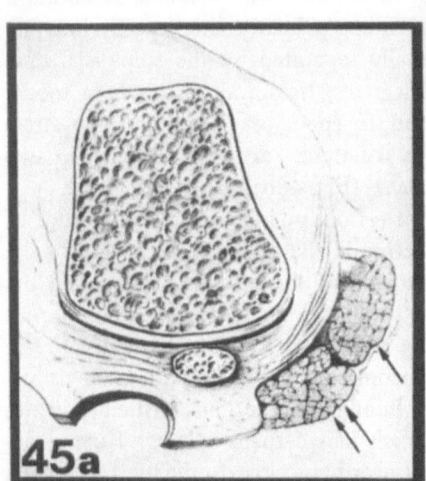

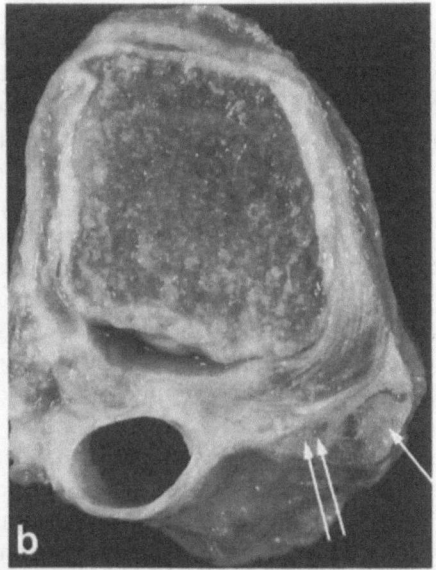

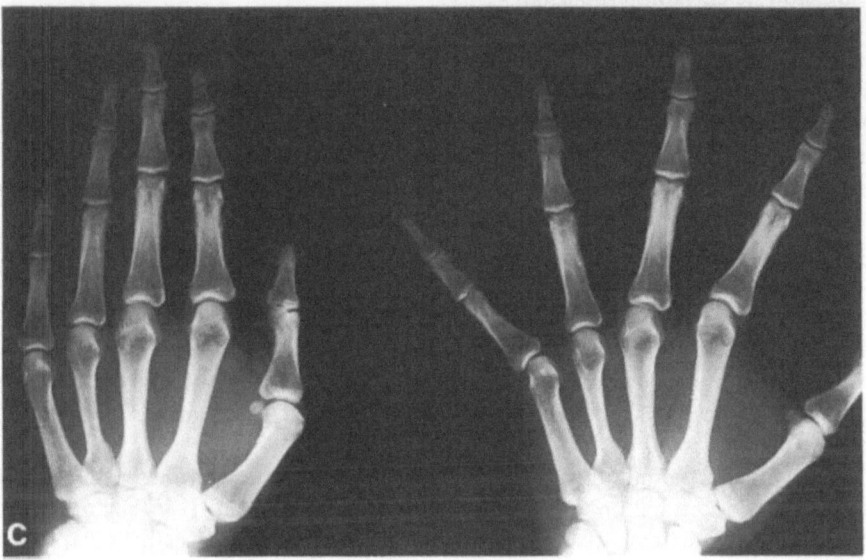

Fig. 45. *a* Section through the right index finger at the point of the metacarpophalangeal joint. The mm. interosseus dorsalis I (*single arrow*) and lumbricalis I (*double arrow*) cross the radial condylus. The palmar fibrous cartilage disk contains a sesamoid bone. Drawing from a sawn section. *b* Section through the left little finger at the point of the metacarpophalangeal joint. The mm. abductor digiti minimi (*single arrow*) and flexor digiti minimi brevis (*double arrow*) cross the ulnar condylus. The joint capsule between muscles and condylus is thickened. *c* Roentgenograms of the left hand of a 35-year-old male proband. On the *left*, fingers II, IV, and V are adducted to the middle finger; on the *right*, abducted maximally

genograms of midsagittal sections through the heads of the ossa metacarpalia II–V show spongiosa extending at right angles from the subchondral compacta. In addition to this, there are two bundles of spongiosa extending palmarly and dorsally into the corticalis of the metaphysis. The two are usually separated by the epiphysial line.

Photoelastic experiments showed the course of stress trajectories in a model of the caput ossis metacarpalis to correspond to spongiosa· structure. The stress trajectories were found to run at right angles from the "articular surface" in two groups towards the area representing the metaphysis (Fig. 46b).

As Kummer (1959) showed for the femur of various young and adult quadrupeds, it may be assumed that the spongiosa architecture in the dorsopalmar region of the caput ossis metacarpalis II–V changes after closure of the growth plate. When the plate is no longer present, the line is bridged and spongiosa forms a continuous pattern, extending into the two columns in the metaphysis. This is particularly clear in cases where the epiphysial line can only be incompletely seen or is not at all visible.

The observation that the dorsal spongiosa bundle is sometimes rarified indicates that pressure on the dorsal part of the caput ossis metacarpalis is lower. Roentgenograms of sagittal sections through the proximal finger bone close to the joint, however, usually show denser dorsal spongiosa.

Cartilage Thickness and Functional Strain. The thickness of articular cartilage is functionally related to the specific strain placed on the joint. Ingelmark and Ekholm (1948) and Ekholm and Ingelmark (1952) were able to record a rapid and reversible increase in the thickness of articular cartilage as a result of experimentally increased stress. Kurrat (1977) and Oberländer (1977) showed that the cartilage layer is thicker in areas of greater stress in the human hip joint. The cartilage was found to be regularly thickest on the caput femoris above the spongiosa bundle that is stressed in compression (Kurrat 1977).

Results of the present study showed the articular cartilage on the metacarpophalangeal joints II–V to be of varying thickness. The thickest area in the joint socket of the first phalanx lay dorsally, while on the metacarpus it was in the palmar part for the ossa metacarpalia II, IV, and V (see Fig. 43). This corresponded to the specific density of the spongiosa.

These findings permit the conclusion that strain is greater on the dorsal part of the oval joint socket and on the palmar region of the metacarpus II–V than otherwise in these joints. In the case of the index finger, the caput ossis metacarpalis was found to be covered with a fairly uniformly thick cartilage layer, permitting the conclusion that the strain is similar in the palmar and central regions.

Examination of the hand in action can help explain the various findings. When a strong grip is required to take hold of a large object, the middle, ring, and little fingers are increasingly bent at the metacarpophalangeal joint. According to Brown (1970) and Hazelton et al. (1975), these fingers provide the necessary retaining strength in a power grip. The thumb, assisted by the nearly extended index finger, provides the precision for the grip. In a three-dimensional stress analysis of the bent metacarpophalangeal joints III–V in a power grip, Chao et al. (1976) calculated the greatest absolute joint stress. Stress on the joints decreases from the middle to the little finger, which corresponds to the reduction in thickness of the subchondral corticalis observed in this study. In the index finger, axial compressive stress on the joint is approximately equal, whether the finger is extended or bent (Chao et al.

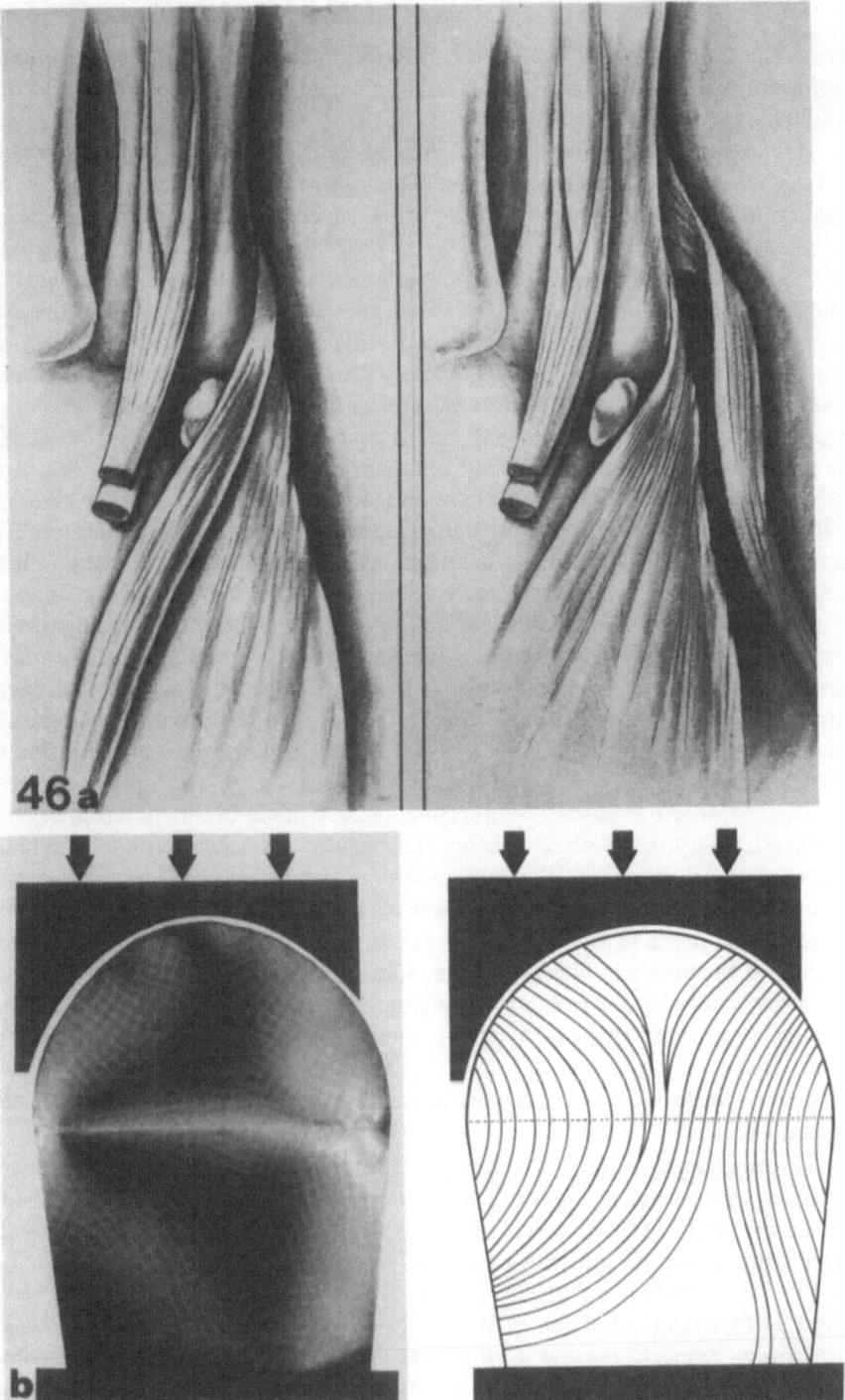

Fig. 46. *a* Position of the sesamoid bone of the index finger, palmar aspect. The m. lumbricalis I partially covers the sesamoid bone (*left*). On the *right*, the muscle is dragged radially; the fibrous cartilage disk has been removed. Drawings from preparations. *b* Course of stress trajectories in a plexiglas model of the caput ossis metacarpalis (*left*) subjected to pressure. On the *right*, the trajectories relevant for this experiment are drawn in

1976). The index finger is bent at the metacarpophalangeal joint for execution of the fingertip or precision grip, for example, to hold a small object between finger and thumb.

This means that the strain on the index finger joint would appear to be about the same in extended and bent positions. This equal strain is reflected in the uniform thickness of the articular cartilage in the palmar and central regions of the metacarpal articular surface.

Cartilage in the dorsal sections of the joint surface of the ossa metacarpalia II—V is thinner than elsewhere. Except in cases of unnatural hyperextension of the meta-carpophalangeal joints, this part of the joint surface does not come into contact with the oval joint socket of the phalanx. The strain stimulus required to retain the cartilage layer (Pauwels 1960) must therefore be provided by the dorsal aponeurosis of the finger extensors, which runs across the metacarpal head and the base of the phalanx, lying on the joint capsule. According to Landsmeer (1955, 1958), Long and Brown (1964), Landsmeer and Long (1965), Smith (1974), and Chao et al. (1976), not only is the aponeurosis dorsalis passively taut when the joints of the fingers are bent, but extensors are also actively contracted. This means they modulate the flexion in the metacarpophalangeal joint and interact with the musculi lumbricales and interossei to retain extension in the middle and tip joints of the fingers (Landsmeer and Long 1965). This permits the conclusion that simultaneous contraction of the flexion muscles and the extensors leads to considerable strain on the metacarpophalangeal joint, particularly of fingers III, IV, and V. This is supported by the arthritic cartilage lesions which were almost exclusively found in the palmar regions of the metacarpal articular surfaces.

The fact that the phalangeal spongiosa is more dense on the dorsal than on the palmar side, the thicker dorsal subchondral compacta, thicker cartilage, and greater frequency of arthritic changes are all indications of the occurrence of maximal strain when the fingers are bent. Such high stress on the dorsal part of the joint socket may be due to the dorsal capsule being taut during flexion. This capsule lies immediately adjacent to the proximal finger bone. In addition to this, Berme et al. (1977) calculated palmar subluxation stress on the phalanx by means of a biomechanical three-dimensional analysis. This stress amounts to about one third of the compressive stress acting axially on the articular surfaces. Contraction of the extensors reduces the subluxation tendency. The dorsal part of the joint socket is pressed against the palmar metacarpal articular surface.

If roentgenograms of bent metacarpophalangeal joints from dissected material are compared with roentgenograms of living probands, the effect of the contracted dorsal aponeurosis becomes clear. In the nonliving material, the joint cleft is dorsally open, which is not the case in the living joints (Fig. 47).

Split Line Patterns and Functional Strain. The split line pattern on the phalangeal joint surface also supports the theory that cartilage is subjected to greater stress in the dorsal part. In many cases, there is an attractive singular point here. According to Tillmann (1971, 1973, 1978) and Molzberger (1973), attractive singular points are found in surface areas where there is high compressive stress. The variable course of the split lines on the distal articular surfaces of the ossa metacarpalia II—V (Stümpel and Koebke in press) seems to be due to the variation in individual strain on the articular surfaces, not only on the dorsopalmar section. Together with the main

68

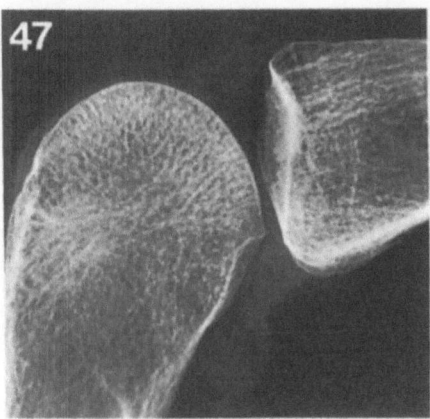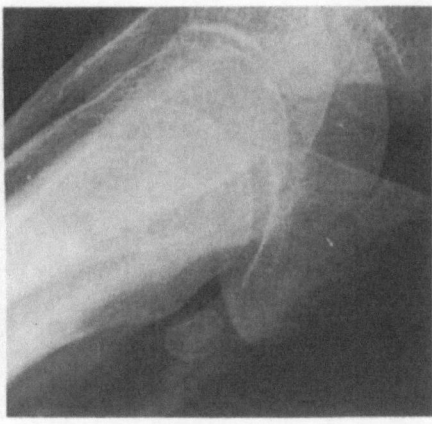

Fig. 47. Side view roentgenogram of the bent metacarpophalangeal index finger joint. *Left*: dissected material; *right*: roentgenogram of living finger

actions of abduction and adduction, and flexion and extension, additional movements involving rotation occur, which vary for the four joints both with regard to the degree and direction of rotation (R. Fick 1904, 1911; Shiino 1925; Landsmeer 1955, 1976; Lewis 1977). Clear proof of correlation between individual split line patterns and strain is hardly possible. In spite of variations, a general basic split line pattern may be discerned (see Fig. 39). This is characterized by a number of parallel lines crossing the dorsopalmar cross-section of the articular surface. They are flanked by a dorsal and palmar radial and ulnar attractive singular points. According to Pauwels (1959), Konermann (1971), and Molzberger (1973), the articular surface represents a "verkörpertes Spannungsfeld", whereby the split line pattern corresponds to the course of stress trajectories in a properly contoured model subjected to similar stress. The collagen fibers of the articular cartilage that will withstand tensile stress run in trajectorial lines in the direction of the greatest tension that may arise under stress (Pauwels 1959).

If a flat, rectangular gelatine model is subjected to uniform pressure, the stress trajectories in the center of the model run in straight lines through the shorter diameter (Pauwels 1959). The surface of the os metacarpale II–V that comes into contact with the smaller oval phalangeal articular surface in positions between extension and 90° flexion roughly corresponds to a biconvexly curved rectangle (Fig. 48). If approximately uniform compressive stress on the articular cartilage may be assumed, as is certainly the case for the metacarpal surface on the index finger, then the course of the split lines seems to refute the experimental findings of this study.

However, if the different sizes of the two articular surfaces are taken into consideration in the model test, so that a rectangular gelatine surface is subjected to pressure by a smaller oval glass plate, then the tension trajectories in the immediate vicinity of the point of pressure run through the smaller diameter of the oval (Fig. 49). When this particular experiment was carried out a few times to imitate the stress placed on the metacarpal articular surface by the smaller phalangeal surface during flexion, the pattern of the tension trajectories ran parallel to the long axis of the rectangular surface. In analogy to the change in direction of the resultant R in the hip joint when the joint is moved, Kummer (1968, 1969) and Tillmann (1969, 1978)

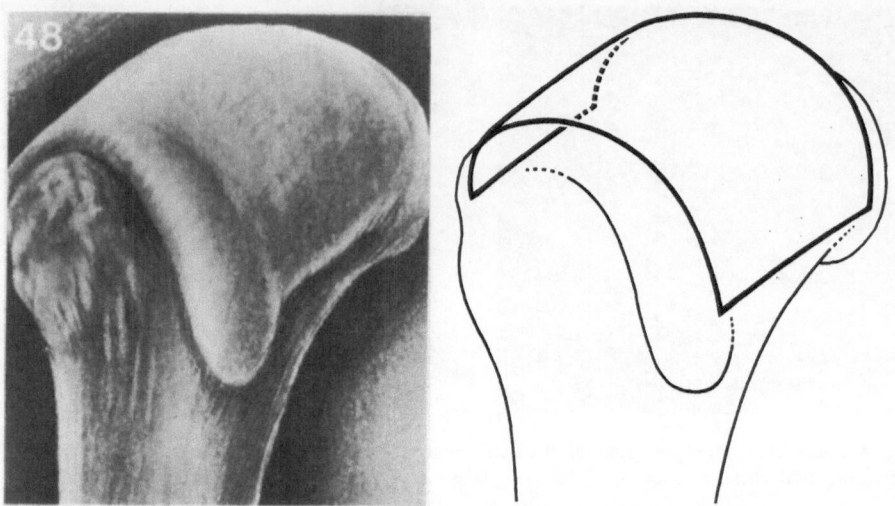

Fig. 48. Sketches of the metacarpal head. The force-transmitting area is comparable to a rectangle, curved biconvexly

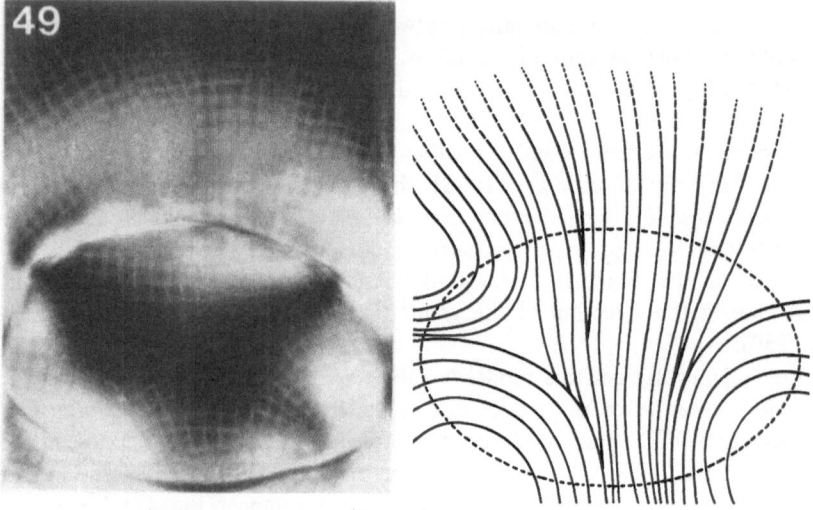

Fig. 49. Course of normal stress trajectories in a gelatine model compressed by an oval glass plate (*left*). On the *right*, the trajectories relevant for this experiment are drawn in

"constructed" the facies lunata of the hip joint socket out of layers of polar caps. In order to fully reproduce the course of the tension trajectories from models of the facies lunata, Molzberger (1973) reconstructed the final experimental result from several individual results. He justified this procedure by indicating that the total articular surface of the facies lunata is composed of several areas submitted separately to strain. As in the hip joint, the momentary zone of cartilage persistence (Tillmann 1969) on the metacarpal articular surface of the metacarpophalangeal joints II–V is smaller than the surface subjected to strain. The entire surface is the result of several overlapping cartilage retention zones due to different strain in different stages of flexion and extension.

Summarizing results for the metacarpophalangeal joints II—V, it would seem that a general plan for all fingers is refined by specific morphological features in the case of each finger. Functional anatomic analysis indicates a clear correlation between the morphological findings and the individual strain placed on the joint in different fingers.

Morphology and Mechanics of the Metacarpophalangeal Thumb Joint. A number of interpretations have been made with regard to form and function of the articulatio metacarphophalangea pollicis. Braus and Elze (1954) considered it to be a restricted ball-and-socket joint, like the other metacarpophalangeal joints, while R. Fick (1904) and Von Lanz and Wachsmuth (1959) held it to be both morphologically and functionally a hinge joint. Strasser (1917) described it as an intermediary form between the interphalangeal and the metacarpophalangeal joints. Measurement of the radioulnar and the dorsopalmar curvature radius of the proximal articular surface led Reimann and Ebner (1980) to the conclusion that the articulatio metacarpophalangea pollicis is egg shaped.

The active degree of flexion in the joint varies individually quite considerably (Parsons 1895; Fick 1911; Harris and Joseph 1949; Joseph 1951a; Reimann and Ebner 1980). According to Joseph (1951a), this is due to the shape of the articular surfaces. Where these are flat, flexion cannot exceed 20°. Where the articular surface is very curved, flexion is said to be possible up to 90° (Parsons 1895). Movement of the first thumb phalanx around a dorsopalmar axis is, according to R. Fick (1911), only passively possible, while Strasser (1917), Bojsen-Møller (1976), and Reimann and Ebner (1980) maintain this is also actively possible. Reimann and Ebner (1980) measured ulnar adduction of 10°—20°. Du Bois-Reymond (1896), Grünkorn (1932), and Braus and Elze (1954) also referred to the possibility of active rotation.

Split Line Patterns, Spongiosa Architecture, and Functional Strain on the Metacarpophalangeal Thumb Joint. Split line analysis of the metacarpal articular surface of thumbs examined here showed a uniform, basic pattern. The split lines were found to run parallel to each other across the center of the articular surface through the dorsopalmar diameter. There were found to be two radial and two ulnar attractive singular points. This pattern corresponds to the basic pattern established for the ossa metacarpalia II—V, except that the central parallel lines now run through the shorter, dorsopalmar diameter of the metacarpal surface. This finding can be explained by the different relationship in the size of the proximal and distal articular surfaces. Especially in cases where the surfaces were rather flat, the phalangeal surface was only slightly smaller than the metacarpal one. Strain on the joint thus results in compressive stress on almost the entire metacarpal articular surface. The direction of the collagen fibers in the tangential layer corresponds to the course of the tension trajectories in a model test where a gelatine surface is compressed by an equally large glass plate (Pauwels 1959).

The relative constancy of the split line pattern on the metacarpal surface of the thumb joint, compared to the high degree of variability found in the patterns for the ossa metacarpalia II—V, indicates uniform distribution of joint strain. Roentgenograms of midsagittal sections of the distal part of the os metacarpale I show strong

71

spongiosa designed for axial pressure. The spongiosa run in two columns into the dorsal and palmar corticalis and are crossed at right angles by the relatively weak spongiosa tension bundles. This permits the conclusion that the main stress on the metacarpophalangeal thumb joint consists of compressive stress on the level of flexion.

Arthrosis of the Metacarpophalangeal Thumb Joint. The degenerative cartilage deficiencies that could be seen on the metacarpal articular surface of 24 of the thumb joints examined were all in the radial part. Cartilage defects are the morphological correlate of localized unphysiologically high strain. In 17 of these thumbs, there was not only cartilage deficiency in the metacarpophalangeal joint but also arthrosis of the thumb saddle joint. Pfiffner (1971), Horvath and Lengyel (1976), and Swanson (1980) reported clinical findings where not only the thumb saddle joint but also other joints near to the os trapezium were affected by arthrosis. Arthrosis of the thumb saddle joint may be expected to have a negative influence on the metacarpophalangeal thumb joint if the typical malpositioning of the thumb occurs, whereby contractive adduction in the thumb saddle joint is combined with hyperextension of the metacarpophalangeal joint. The contractive adduction leads to a pathological increase in joint pressure in

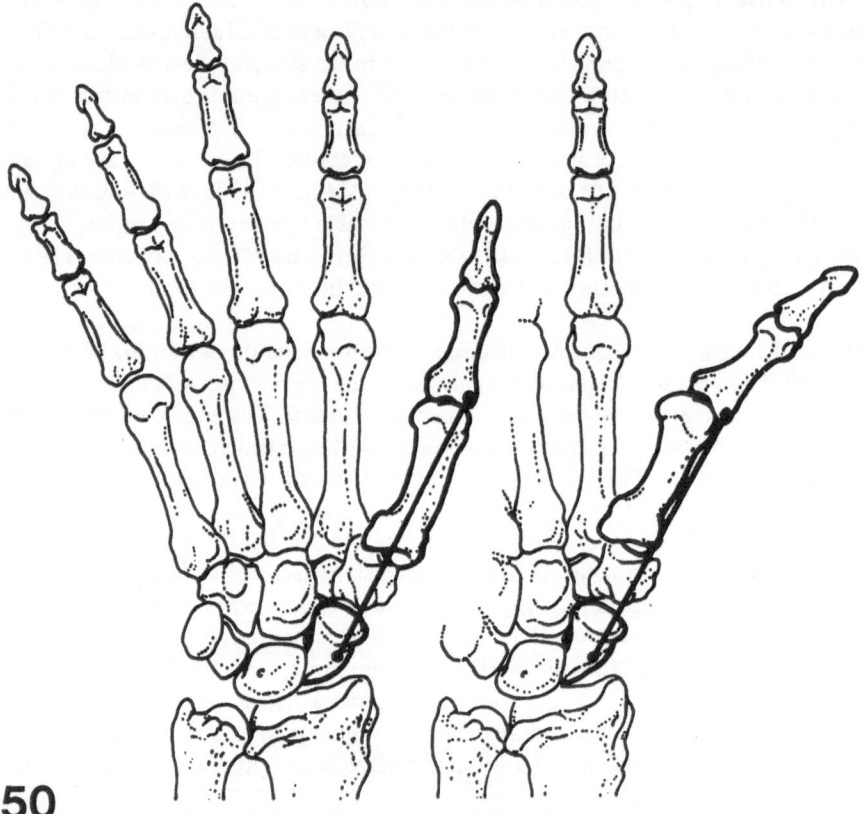

50

Fig. 50. Course of the main line of the m. abductor pollicis brevis from the os scaphoideum to the base of the first phalanx. In the healthy thumb (*left*), the muscle bends the thumb in the metacarpophalangeal joint. Malpositioning of adduction in the thumb saddle joint (*right*) alters the course of the muscle to such an extent that it extends and causes abduction

the palmar and ulnar regions (Koebke and Thomas 1979a, b) and causes local cartilage lesions. The findings of this study indicate that the dorsal and radial areas of the meta-carpal articular surface in the metacarpophalangeal thumb joint are subjected to ex-cessive stress.

It has been said that the malpositioning in adduction of the thumb saddle joint is due to contraction of the musculus adductor pollicis (Swanson 1980). If a reason for the malpositioning of the metacarpophalangeal joint is to be sought, it is mis-leading to refer to this as compensatory hyperextension (Pfiffner 1971). It should rather be seen as necessarily concurrent with malpositioning of the thumb saddle joint. Landsmeer (1961a, b, 1976) showed that three sets of muscles are necessary for coordinated movement of a chain with three links connected by two joints. In the four fingers, these three muscle sets are the extensors, the long flexors, and the mm. lumbricales and interossei. The relative positioning of the muscles to the axis of the metacarpophalangeal and middle joints of the finger determines the effect the individual muscles have on the joint and makes it possible, for example, to bend both joints simultaneously. Malfunctioning or poor alignment of the central line of any of these muscles disrupts the system and leads to the so-called zigzag position of the middle link of the chain (Landsmeer 1976).

If this principle is transferred to the joints of the thumb, the m. abductor pollicis brevis would seem to occupy a key position. During contracted adduction of the thumb saddle joint, the main tension line of this muscle moves radiodorsally. Its side insertion at the radial base of the phalanx means that the muscle no longer leads to flexion in the metacarpophalangeal joint, but to extension and abduction (Fig. 50). The muscle pulls the first phalanx into this malposition and retains it there.

In summary, the metacarpophalangeal thumb joint gives evidence of functional adaptations typical of a hinge joint. The main source of joint strain is through com-pressive stress during flexion. Abduction, adduction, and rotation cannot be excluded as secondary movements.

Rhizarthrosis and the simultaneous malpositioning of the metacarpophalangeal thumb joint require conservative or sometimes even operative therapy (Swanson 1980). The function of the m. abductor pollicis brevis should not be forgotten when causal therapy is being considered.

5 General Conclusion

The fundamental concept of biomechanics is based upon the scientific investigations of Pauwels (summarized in 1965). He was the first to clarify the more speculative hypothesis of Roux (1895) concerning functional adaptation, especially of the human skeleton system. In Roux's (1895) theory, each bone is adapted to the actual mechan-ical stress acting on it and functions on the basis of the "maximum-minimum law." Accordingly, many authors investigated bones and joints of the human skeleton in order to prove the hypothesis that, in general, the amount and the structure of skeletal material is related to its specific mechanical stress.

Several biomechanical methods (newly introduced by Pauwels 1965) are applic-able to these studies. With the aid of the photoelastic method, it is possible to analyze the distribution of stress or the direction of stress trajectories in models of bones or joints. It has been shown by Kummer (1959) that the results of photoelastic experiments, i.e., the mode of distribution or direction of stress, are transferable to bones or joints. Investigation of the architecture of trabecular bone by roentgenography and determination of the density of bone substance with equidenses are useful to demonstrate relations between the physiological strain and the distribution and density of spongy or compact bone. Furthermore, the distribution of pressure within a cartilaginous articular surface can be analyzed by the split line method. Combined with photoelastic experiments, this method allows deductions to be made about the pattern of strain on each individual articular surface. Such biomechanical investigations, especially of the joints of the lower limb, have laid the ground for causal therapy in many cases of joint diseases (Pauwels 1935, 1961, 1976; Maquet 1976). These studies demonstrate that a given overloading of a restricted area of a joint results in a degeneration of cartilage and bone. However, after reduction of the state of overloading by orthopedic surgery, the joint will recover. Thus, bone and cartilage specifically react to mechanical stimuli.

The present investigation on the proximal wrist joint, the saddle joint of the thumb, and the metacarpophalangeal joints demonstrates that these joints are adapted to their specific function. The discus articularis on the ulnar side of the proximal wrist joint is of great importance for normal hand functions. Degeneration of the disk, mechanical in origin, may lead to incongruency of joint surfaces and severe disturbance of joint function.

The saddle joint of the thumb under physiological conditions is subject to strain typical for a ball-and-socket joint. Opposing the thumb, the os metacarpale I rotates and reduces the pressure-transmitting area in the joint. Cases of arthrosis are in all likelihood rooted in the increase of mechanical stress due to incongruency of articular surfaces.

The size and shape of the metacarpophalangeal joints, as well as the thickness of cartilage and the distribution of bone material within the metacarpal heads, strongly suggest a very specific adaptation of each finger to individual function.

6 Summary

The present study attempts to show the relationship between morphology and normal or defective functioning, as demonstrated by three joints that play an important role in the use of the human hand. To this end, the articulatio radiocarpea, the articulatio carpometacarpea pollicis, and the articulationes metacarpophalangeae are analyzed from a functional anatomic point of view. Macroscopic, microscopic anatomic, and histological examinations are carried out on material from the dissection rooms. Split line techniques are used to trace the course of collagen fibers in the tangential fiber layer of the articular cartilage, and roentgenographic examination and equidensity methods permit conclusions to be drawn about the structure and density of the bone material. Joint strain is evaluated by comparing the morphological findings with the results of photoelastic model tests. The transfer of energy from the upper arm to the forearm is experimentally analyzed with the help of prepared material subjected to dynamic stress.

The focal point of the examination of the *articulatio radiocarpea* is the discus articularis. When the hand and arm are used, this disk transfers compressive stress between caput ulnae and os lunatum. This view is supported by histological findings and by the analysis of the tangential fiber layer of the articular cartilage. The frequently observed perforation of the disk may be attributed to the high mechanical strain from compressive load. Perforation of the disk is frequently followed by arthritic cartilage deficiencies on the os lunatum and the caput ulnae.

Experimental studies with arms from the dissection room show that the articular disk is frequently damaged when the radius is fractured in the classical fashion. Classical fracture of the radius can also be induced when the membrana interossea has previously been severed. This is interpreted to mean that this membrane – contrary to the view usually expressed in the literature – plays no major part in the transfer of energy between the bones of the forearm. Experimental evidence indicates that both bones are subjected directly to compressive stress. In this case the discus articularis functions as a cushion for the ulna. Further measurement on arms subjected to dynamic load indicates that the membrana interossea antebrachii plays only a minor role in energy transfer from the upper arm to the hand. In the neutral central position and in pronation with the hand in dorsal extension and radial abduction, more than 80% of the energy is transferred via the radius, irrespective of whether the membrane is intact or not. With increasing supination, the amount of energy transmitted by the ulna rises.

The results of examination of the *articulatio carpometacarpea pollicis* give indications of the etiology and genesis of arthrosis of the thumb saddle joint (rhizarthrosis). The position of cartilage lesions on the two articular surfaces indicates rotation in the joint during oppositional movement of the thumb. The rotation leads to incongruency of the joint with only spot contact between the articular surfaces. These findings are retraced in photoelastic experiments, and it can be shown that stress peaks occur together with incongruency. This leads to the conclusion that the extreme reduction in the surface area for transmission of forces during opposition causes stress peaks on the articular surfaces of the joint. The defects in the articular cartilage are seen as the morphological correlate of a mechanical overloading of the cartilage and as the first stage of rhizarthrosis.

Analysis of the course of the collagen fibers in the tangential fiber layer of the articular cartilage on the os trapezium and the os metacarpale I support this theory. The cartilage is functionally adapted to the distribution of stress that may be expected to arise during the execution of normal movements of a saddle joint – abduction, adduction, flexion, and extension. The cartilage gives no evidence of being suited to the high local pressure that arises in conjunction with joint incongruency due to rotational movement during opposition.

Examination of the capsular ligaments shows that the ligamentum metacarpeum dorsale I between the os metacarpale II and the capsule of the thumb saddle joint plays a key role in the function of the joint. Normally, the ligament prevents radial luxation of the thumb. Preparatoy, histological, and roentgenographic findings indicate that there is a correlation between overloading of this ligament and the development of rhizarthrosis. The formation of a spur at the base of the os metacarpale II is due to partial ossification of the ligament. This appears to be caused by an increase in radial tension. The ligament is stretched too far and the thumb takes up a radial malposition that is typical of advanced arthrosis of the thumb saddle joint.

The shape of the joint members and the architecture of the spongiosa are investigated on the *articulationes metacarpophalangeae*. The split line method permits the direction of the collagen fibers in the tangential fiber layer of the articular cartilage to be analyzed, while equidensity examination shows the distribution of density of the bone material in the subchondral compacta. The findings obtained permit the conclusion that the individual joints are characterized by specific morphological features corresponding to the particular function of the finger. Macroscopic findings for the metacarpophalangeal joint of the thumb seem to indicate a causal relationship between lesions of the articular cartilage on the caput ossis metacarpalis I and arthrosis in the thumb saddle joint.

Acknowledgements. The author gratefully acknowledges Prof. Dr. B. Tillmann and Prof. Dr. H. Leonhardt for their suggestions and criticism. Thanks are due to Miss U. Kruse for her skillful technical assistance and to Mr. R. Clemens for drawing several figures.

7 References

Adler H (1975) Zur Frage der normalen Stabilität des Daumensattelgelenks. Handchirurgie 7:115–116

Altmann K (1964) Zur kausalen Histogenese des Knorpels. W Roux's Theorie und die experimentelle Wirklichkeit. Ergeb Anat Entwicklungsgesch 44:1–167

Anderson RJ (1901) Rotation of the forearm. Lancet 2:1333–1334

Arendt W (1955) Über das distale Radio-Ulnargelenk. Beitr Orthop Traumatol Sonderheft 2:101–114

Aune S (1955) Oesteo-arthritis in the first carpo-metacarpal joint. Acta Chir Scand 109:449–456

Backhouse KM, Catton WT (1954) An experimental study of the functions of the lumbrical muscles in the human hand. J Anat 88:133–141

Barnett CH, Davies DV, Mac Conaill MA (1961) Synovial joints. Their structure and mechanics. Longmans, London

Bausenhardt D (1949/50) Über das Carpo-Metacarpalgelenk des Daumens. Z Anat Entwicklungsgesch 114:251–256

Becker W, Krahl H (1978) Die Tendopathien. Thieme, Stuttgart

Bergerhoff W (1944) Über die Normung der Röntgenaufnahmen. Roentgenpraxis 16:37–47

Bergk K, Thümler P (1979) Das Daumensattelgelenk – Schlüsselgelenk des Daumens. Verh Anat Ges 73:173–180

Berme N, Paul JP, Purves WK (1977) A biomechanical analysis of the metacarpophalangeal joint. J Biomech 10:409–412

Blauth W, Schneider-Sickert F (1976) Handfehlbildungen. Springer, Berlin Heidelberg New York

Böhler J (1969) Gelenknahe Frakturen des Unterarms. Chirurg 40:198–203

Bojsen-Møller F (1976) Osteoligamentous guidance of the movements of the human thumb. Am J Anat 147:71–80

Bopp HM (1965) Anatomische Untersuchungen der Daumensattelgelenksarthrose. Inauguraldissertation Köln

Brade A, Koebke J (1979) Probleme bei veralteten distalen Radiusfrakturen. Orthop Prax 9:727–729

Brade A, Koebke J (in press) Experimentell erzeugte distale Radiusfrakturen. Z Orthop

Braithwaite F, Channell G, Moore F, Whillis J (1948) The applied anatomy of the lumbrical and interosseous muscles of the hand. Guy's Hosp Rep 97:185–195

Braune W (1887) Über den Mechanismus der menschlichen Hand. Anat Anz 2:395–396

Braus H (1954) Anatomie des Menschen. Ein Lehrbuch für Studierende und Ärzte. Fortgeführt von Elze C, vol I, Bewegungsapparat, 3rd edn. Springer, Berlin Göttingen Heidelberg

Brösike G (1892) Cursus der normalen Anatomie des menschlichen Körpers, 3rd edn. Fischers Medicinische Buchhandlung, Berlin

Brown HG (1970) Functional anatomy of the hand. Orthop Clin North Am 1:199—204

Bunnel S (1938) Opposition of the thumb. J Bone Joint Surg 20:269—284

Carlsöö S, Johansson O (1962) Stabilization of and load on the elbow joint in some protective movements. An experimental study. Acta Anat (Basel) 48:224—231

Cathcart CW (1885) On the movements of the ulna in pronation and supination. J Anat Physiol 19:355—362

Chao EY, Opgrande JD, Axmear FE (1976) Three-dimensional force analysis of the finger joints in selected isometric hand functions. J Biomech 9:387—396

Coleman HM (1960) Injuries of the articular disc at the wirst. J Bone Joint Surg 42 B:522—529

Corner E (1898) The morphology of the triangular cartilage of the wrist. J Anat 32:272—274

Corrucini R (1977) Features of the prosimian wrist joint in relation to hominoid specializations. Acta Anat (Basel) 99:440—444

Cotta H, Mittelmeier H (1959) Die Arthrose der Handwurzel. Z Orthop 91:567—582

Dahhan P, Fischer L, Allieu Y (1980) The trapezio-metacarpal articulation. Anat clin 2:43—56

De La Caffinière JY (1970) L'articulation trapézo-métacarpienne. Approche biomécanique et appareil ligamentaire. Arch Anat Cytol Pathol 18:277—284

De Palma AF (1957) Degenerative changes in the sternoclavicular and acromioclavicular joints in various decades. Thomas, Springfield

De Seze S, Ryckewaert A (1954) Maladies des os et des articulations. Flammarion, Paris

Destot E, Gallois E (1896) Recherches physiologiques et expérimentales sur les fractures de l'extrémité inférieure du radius (radiographie). Rev Chir Orthop 18:886—915

Du Bois-Reymond R (1895) Über das Sattelgelenk. Arch Anat Physiol Physiol Abt 5/6:433—462

Du Bois-Reymond R (1896) Die Gelenkbewegungen bei der Opposition. Anat Anz 11:464—467

Duchenne GB (1949) Physiology of movement. Lippincott, Philadelphia

Duparc J, De La Caffinière JY, Pineau H (1971) Approche bio-mécanique et cotation des mouvements du premier métacarpien. Rev Chir Orthop 57:3—12

Dwight T (1885) The movements of the ulna in rotation of the forearm. J Anat Physiol 19:186—189

Eaton R, Littler J (1969) A study of the basal joint of the thumb. Treatment of its disabilities by fusion. J Bone Joint Surg 51A:661—668

Ekholm R, Ingelmark BE (1952) Functional thickness variations of human articular cartilage. Acta Soc Med Ups 57:39—59

Faller A (1980) Anatomie in Stichworten. Enke, Stuttgart

Ferber Ch (1953) Ein Beitrag zur Dreigliedrigkeit des „Daumens." Z Orthop 83:55—64

Fick A (1854) Die Gelenke mit sattelförmigen Flächen. Z rat Med NF 4:314—321

Fick R (1904) Handbuch der Anatomie des Menschen, vol 2, pt I, I, Anatomie der Gelenke. Fischer, Jena

Fick R (1911) Handbuch der Anatomie des Menschen, vol 2, pt I, 3, Spezielle Gelenk- und Muskelmechanik. Fischer, Jena

Fischer O (1897) Ueber Gelenke von zwei Graden der Freiheit. Arch Anat Physiol Anat Abt Suppl 242—272

Fischer O (1907) Kinematik organischer Gelenke. Vieweg, Braunschweig

Fischer O (1919) Medizinische Physik, 2nd edn. Hirzel, Leipzig

Flatt AE (1974) The care of the rheumatoid hand, 3rd edn. Mosby, Saint Louis

Flower WH (1885) An introduction to the osteology of the mammalia, 3rd edn. Macmillan, London

Föppl L, Mönch E (1950) Praktische Spannungsoptik. Springer, Berlin Göttingen Heidelberg

Forestier J (1937) L'ostéo-arthrite sèche trapézo-métacarpienne. Presse méd 45:315—317

Frykman G (1967) Fracture of the distal radius including sequelae-shoulder-hand-finger syndrome, disturbance in the distal radio-ulnar joint and impairment of nerve function. A clinical and experimental study. Acta Orthop Scand [Suppl] 108:1—153

Gegenbaur C (1895) Lehrbuch der Anatomie des Menschen, vol I, 6th edn. Engelmann, Leipzig

Geschwend N (1970) L'arthrose de l'articulation basale du pouce ou rhizarthrose du pouce et son traitement opératoire. Méd hyg 944:1971—1973

Golden GN (1963) Treatment and prognosis of Colles' fracture. Lancet 1:511—515

Gräfenberg E (1914) Die entwicklungsgeschichtliche Bedeutung der Hyperdaktylie menschlicher Gliedmaßen. Stud Path Entw 2:565–589

Grünkorn J (1932) Die Daumenopposition, ihre muskelphysiologische Erklärung und die Behandlung des Oppositionsausfalls. (Unter besonderer Berücksichtigung der v. Baeyerschen Sehnentranslokation). Z Orthop Chir 57:430–517

Günther G (1850) Das Handgelenk. Hamburg

Guyot J (1981) Atlas of human limb joints. Springer, Berlin Heidelberg New York

Haage H (1966) Die Arthrografie des Handgelenks. I. Mitt. Das normale Gelenk und seine Variationen. Radiologe 6:50–57

Haage H (1973) Arthrografie des Handgelenks. In: Diethelm L, Olsson O, Strand F, Vieten H, Zuppinger A (eds) Handbuch der Medizinischen Radiologie, vol 5/2. Springer, Berlin Heidelberg New York, pp 353–398

Haage H, Cornelius H (1966) Die Arthrografie des Handgelenks. II. Mitt. Der pathologische Discus articularis. Radiologe 6:58–63

Hackenbroch M (1943) Die Arthrosis deformans der Hüfte. Grundlagen und Behandlung. Thieme, Leipzig

Haines RW (1944) The mechanism of rotation at the first carpo-metacarpal joint. J Anat 78:44–46

Halls A, Travill A (1964) Transmission of pressures across the elbow joint. Anat Rec 150:243–248

Harris HA (1934) Calcification and ossification in the semilunar cartilages. Lancet 1:1114–1116

Harris H, Joseph J (1949) Variation in extension of the metacarpophalangeal and interphalangeal joints of the thumb. J Bone Joint Surg 31:547–559

Hazelton FT, Smidt GL, Flatt AE, Stephens RJ (1975) The influence of wrist position on the force produced by the finger flexors. J Biomech 8:301–306

Heiberg J (1885) The movements of the ulna in rotation of the fore-arm. J Anat Physiol 19:237–240

Heitzmann C (1875) Die descriptive und topografische Anatomie des Menschen, vol I, 2nd edn. Braumüller, Wien

Helbig B, Steinbach M (1978) Bemerkungen zur operativen Behandlung der Daumensattelgelenksarthrose. Schleswig-Holsteinisches Ärztebl 3:185–189

Henckel KO (1931) Beitrag zur Entwicklung der Primatenhand. III. Über die Entstehung des Discus articularis des distalen Radio-Ulnargelenkes beim Menschen. Morph Jb 68:293–300

Henke J (1863) Handbuch der Anatomie und Mechanik der Gelenke mit Rücksicht auf Luxationen und Contracturen. Winter'sche Verlagsbuchhandlung, Heidelberg

Henle J (1855) Handbuch der systematischen Anatomie des Menschen, vol 1, pt I, Knochenlehre. Vieweg, Braunschweig

Hirsch D, Page D, Miller D, Dumbleton JH, Miller EH (1974) A biomechanical analysis of the metacarpophalangeal joint of the thumb. J Biomech 7:343–348

Hoegen K, Reske W (1956) Veränderungen an der dreieckigen Bandscheibe des distalen Radio-Ulnar-Gelenks. (Ein Beitrag zur Klinik und Pathologie). Z Orthop 87:525–532

Hofmann S (1959) Der Bau des Discus articularis articulationis radio-ulnaris distalis. Anat Anz 106:173–184

Horváth F, Lengyel E (1976) Arthrose des 1. Strahles der Hand bei geriatrischem Krankengut. Z Orthop 114:822–827

Hultkrantz W (1898) Über die Spaltrichtungen der Gelenkknorpel. Verh Anat Ges 12:248–256

Hyrtl J (1885) Lehrbuch der Anatomie des Menschen. Mit Rücksicht auf physiologische Begründung und praktische Anwendung. Braumüller, Wien

Ingelmark BE, Ekholm R (1948) A study on variations in the thickness of articular cartilage in association with rest and periodical load. An experimental investigation on rabbits. 'Acta Soc Med Ups 53:61–74

Joseph J (1951a) Further studies of the metacarpo-phalangeal and interphalangeal joints of the thumb. J Anat 85:221–229

Joseph J (1951b) The sesamoid bones of the hand and the time of fusion of the epiphysis of the thumb. J Anat 85:230–241

Kapandji A (1963) Schémas commentés de mécanique articulaire. Presse méd 71:1581–1584

Kapandji A (1972) La rotation du pouce sur son axe longitudinal lors de l'opposition. Étude géométrique et mécanique de la trapézo-métacarpienne (modèle mécanique de la main). Rev Chir Orthop 58:273–289

Kaplan E (1966) The participation of the metacarpophalangeal joint of the thumb in the act of opposition. Bull Hosp Joint Dis 27:39–45

Kauer JMG (1975) The articular disc of the hand. Acta Anat (Basel) 93:590–605

Kessler J, Silberman Z (1961) An experimental study of the radiocarpal joint by arthrography. Surg Gynecol Obstet 112:33–40

Klein W, Huth F (1980) Arthroskopie und Histologie von Kniegelenkserkrankungen. Schattauer, Stuttgart

Knief JJ (1967) Materialverteilung und Beanspruchungsverteilung im coxalen Femurende. Densitometrische und spannungsoptische Untersuchungen. Z Anat Entwicklungsgesch 126:81–116

Koebke J (1980) Anatomische Befunde an Händen mit triphalangem Daumen. Handchirurgie 12:219–223

Koebke J, Brade A (1980) Zur Läsion des Discus articularis des Handgelenks. Z Orthop 118:616

Koebke J, Stümpel E (1981) Untersuchungen zu einer Funktionsanalyse der Metacarpophalangealgelenke II–V der menschlichen Hand. Verh Anat Ges 75:275–276

Koebke J, Thomas W (1979a) Biomechanische Untersuchungen zur Ätiologie der Daumensattelgelenksarthrose. Z Orthop 117:988–994

Koebke J, Thomas W (1979b) Funktionell-morphologische Untersuchungen zur Daumensattelgelenksarthrose. Verh Anat Ges 73:181–184

Koebke J, Tillmann B (1977) Zur funktionellen Beanspruchung des Processus styloideus. Verh Anat Ges 71:1289–1296

Köhler A, Zimmer A (1953) Grenzen des Normalen und Anfänge des Pathologischen im Röntgenbilde des Skeletts. Thieme, Stuttgart

Konermann H (1971) Funktionelle Analyse der Knorpelstruktur des Talo-Naviculargelenkes. Z Anat Entwicklungsgesch 133:1–36

Krmpotić-Nemanić J (1967) Über einen bisher unbeachteten Mechanismus der Fingergrundgelenke. Gegenseitige Längsverschiebung der Finger bei der Flexion. Z Anat Entwicklungsgesch 126:127–131

Krompecher St (1937) Die Knochenbildung. Fischer, Jena

Kuczynski K (1974) Carpometacarpal joint of the human thumb. J Anat 118:119–126

Küsswetter W (1979) Einfluß der Membrana interossea antebrachii auf die Umwendbewegung der Hand. Fortschr Med 97:1505–1508

Küsswetter W (1981) Morphologie und Biomechanik der Membrana interossea antebrachii. Thieme, Stuttgart

Küsswetter W, Kibler Th (1977) Biomechanische Untersuchungen zur operativen Behandlung bei Dislokation der Ulna im distalen Radioulnargelenk. Z Orthop 115:941–948

Kummer B (1956) Eine vereinfachte Methode zur Darstellung von Spannungstrajektorien, gleichzeitig ein Modellversuch für die Ausrichtung und Dichteverteilung der Spongiosa in den Gelenkenden der Röhrenknochen. 8. Beitrag zur funktionellen Anatomie und kausalen Morphologie des Stützapparates von Friedrich Pauwels. Z Anat Entwicklungsgesch 119:223–234

Kummer B (1959) Bauprinzipien des Säugerskelettes. Thieme, Stuttgart

Kummer B (1962) Funktioneller Bau und funktionelle Anpassung des Knochens. Anat Anz 111:261–293

Kummer B (1968) Die Beanspruchung des menschlichen Hüftgelenks. I. Allgemeine Problematik. Z Anat Entwicklungsgesch 127:277–285

Kummer B (1969) Die Beanspruchung der Gelenke, dargestellt am Beispiel des menschlichen Hüftgelenks. Enke, Stuttgart, pp 301–311

Kummer B (1975) Biomechanik der Gelenke (Diarthrosen). Die Beanspruchung des Gelenkknorpels. Biopolymere und Biomechanik von Bindegewebssystemen. Z Wiss Konf Deutsch Nat Forsch Ärzte. Springer, Berlin Heidelberg New York

Kummer B (1978) Anatomie fonctionelle et biomécanique de la hanche. Acta Orthop Belg 44:94–104

Kurrat H (1977) Die Beanspruchung des menschlichen Hüftgelenks. VI. Eine funktionelle Analyse der Knorpeldickenverteilung am menschlichen Femurkopf. Anat Embryol (Berl) 150:129–140

Laarmann A (1956) Die chirurgischen Berufskrankheiten. Enke, Stuttgart

Landsmeer J (1955) Anatomical and functional investigations on the articulation of the human fingers. Acta Anat (Basel) 25:Suppl 24, 1–69

Landsmeeer J (1958) A report of the co-ordination of the interphalangeal joints of the human finger and its disturbances. Acta Morphol Neerl Scand 2:59–84

Landsmeer J (1961a) Studies in the anatomy of articulation. I. The equilibrium of the intercalated bone. Acta Morphol Neerl Scand 3:287–303

Landsmeer J (1961b) Studies in the anatomy of articulation. I. Patterns of movement of bi-muscular, bi-articular systems. Acta Morphol Neerl Scand 3:304–321

Landsmeer J (1962) Power grip and precision handling. Ann Rheum Dis 21:164–170

Landsmeer J (1976) Atlas of anatomy of the hand. Churchill Livingstone, Edinburgh

Landsmeer J, Ansingh HR (1957) X-ray observations of rotation of the fingers in the metacarpophalangeal joints. Acta Anat (Basel) 30:404–410

Landsmeer J, Long C (1965) The mechanism of finger control, based on electromyograms and location analysis. Acta Anat (Basel) 60:330–347

Lang F (1942) Das distale Radioulnargelenk. Monatsschr Unfallheilkd Beiheft 36:1–85

Leboucq H (1886) Sur la morphologie du carpe et du tarse. Anat Anz 1:17–21

Lewis OJ (1965) Evolutionary change in the primate wrist and inferior radio-ulnar joints. Anat Rec 151:275–286

Lewis OJ (1970) The development of the human wrist joint during the fetal period. Anat Rec 166:499–516

Lewis OJ (1972) Osteological features characterizing the wrists of monkeys and apes, with a reconstruction of this region in *Dryopithecus africanus*. Am J Phys Antrophol 36:45–58

Lewis OJ (1977) Joint remodelling and the evolution of the human hand. J Anat 123:157–201

Lewis OJ, Hamshere RJ, Bucknill TM (1970) The anatomy of the wrist joint. J Anat 106:539–552

Lewis RM (1950) Colles'-fracture – causative mechanism. Surgery 27:427–434

Long C, Brown ME (1964) Electromyographic kinesiology of the hand: muscles moving the long finger. J Bone Joint Surg 46A:1683–1706

Mac Conaill MA (1931/32) The function of intra-articular fibrocartilages, with special references to the knee and inferior radio-ulnar joints. J Anat 66:210–227

Mac Conaill MA (1946) Studies in the mechanics of synovial joints. II. Displacements on articular surfaces and the significance of saddle joints. Ir J Med Sci July:223–235

Mannerfeld L (1978) Über die möglichen Ursachen der Daumensattelgelenksarthrose. Z Orthop 116:459

Maquet P (1976) Biomechanics of the knee. Springer, Berlin Heidelberg New York

Mason ML (1954) Observations on fractures of the head of the radius with a review of one hundred cases. Br J Surg 42:123–132

Martinek H (1977) Zur Traumatologie des Discus articularis des Handgelenks. 1. Teil: Klinik und Diagnostik. Arch Orthop Unfallchir 87:285–297

Mayfield JK, Johnson RP, Kilcoyne RF (1976) The ligaments of the human wrist and their functional significance. Anat Rec 186:417–428

Meyer H (1873) Die Statik und Mechanik des menschlichen Knochengerüsts. Engelmann, Leipzig

Mikić Ž (1978) Age changes in the triangular fibrocartilage of the wrist joint. J Anat 126:367–384

Mörike K (1964) Zur Herkunft und Funktion des ulnaren Diskus am Handgelenk. Morph Jb 105:365–374

Molzberger H (1973) Die Beanspruchung des menschlichen Hüftgelenks. IV. Analyse der funktionellen Struktur der Tangentialfaserschicht des Hüftpfannenknorpels. Z Anat Entwicklungsgesch 139:283–306

Müller G (1949) Arthrodesis of the trapezio-metacarpal joint for osteoarthritis. J Bone Joint Surg 31B:540–542

Müller W (1937) Die angeborenen Fehlbildungen der menschlichen Hand. Thieme, Leipzig

Napier JR (1955) The form and function of the carpo-metacarpal joint of the thumb. J Anat 89:362–369

Napier JR (1956) The prehensile movements of the human hand. J Bone Joint Surg 38B:902–913

Napier JR, Napier PH (1967) A handbook of living primates. Morphology, ecology and behaviour of non-human primates. Academic, London

Niessen H (1934) Untersuchungen über die Zwischenknorpel der Gelenke. Arch Orthop Unfallchir 34:495–529

Nicolić V, Hančević J, Hudec M, Banović B (1975) Absorption of the impact energy in the palmar soft tissues. Anat Embryol (Berl) 148:215–221

Oberländer W (1977) Die Beanspruchung des menschlichen Hüftgelenks. VII. Die Verteilung der Knorpeldicke im Acetabulum und ihre funktionelle Deutung. Anat Embryol (Berl) 150: 141–153

Oberländer W (1978) Über den Einfluß der funktionellen Knorpelquellung auf die Mechanik kongruenter Gelenke. Verh Anat Ges 72:157–162

Olivier G (1962) Formation du squelette des membres chez l'homme. Vigot, Paris

Parsons FG (1895) On the movements of the metacarpo-phalangeal joint of the thumb. J Anat Physiol 29:446–452

Parsons FG (1900) The joints of mammals compared with those of man. J Anat 34:41–68

Pauwels F (1935) Der Schenkelhalsbruch. Ein mechanisches Problem. Grundlagen des Heilungs-vorganges. Prognose und kausale Therapie. Z Orthop Unfallchir 63:Beilageheft

Pauwels F (1948) Die Bedeutung der Bauprinzipien des Stütz- und Bewegungsapparates für die Beanspruchung der Röhrenknochen. 1. Beitrag zur funktionellen Anatomie und kausalen Morphologie des Stützapparates. Z Anat Entwicklungsgesch 114:129–166

Pauwels F (1955) Über die Verteilung der Spongiosadichte im coxalen Femurende und ihre Be-deutung für die Lehre vom funktionellen Bau des Knochens. 7. Beitrag zur funktionellen Anatomie und kausalen Morphologie des Stützapparates. Morph Jb 95:33–54

Pauwels F (1959) Die Struktur der Tangentialfaserschicht des Gelenkknorpels der Schulterpfanne als Beispiel für ein verkörpertes Spannungsfeld. 9. Beitrag zur funktionellen Anatomie und kausalen Morphologie des Stützapparates. Z Anat Entwicklungsgesch 121:188–240

Pauwels F (1960) Eine neue Theorie über den Einfluß mechanischer Reize auf die Differenzierung des Stützgewebe. 10. Beitrag zur funktionellen Anatomie und kausalen Morphologie des Stützapparates. Z Anat Entwicklungsgesch 121:478–515

Pauwels F (1961) Neue Richtlinien für die operative Behandlung der Koxarthrose. Ver Dtsch Orthop Ges 48. Kongr., pp 232–266

Pauwels F (1963) Die Druckverteilung im Ellenbogengelenk, nebst grundsätzlichen Bemerkungen über den Gelenkdruck. 11. Beitrag zur funktionellen Anatomie und kausalen Morphologie des Stützapparates. Z Anat Entwicklungsgesch 123:643–667

Pauwels F (1965) Gesammelte Abhandlungen zur Biomechanik des Bewegungsapparates. Springer, Berlin Heidelberg New York

Pauwels F (1968) Der Platz der Osteotomie in der operativen Behandlung der Coxarthrose. Triangle 8:196–210

Pauwels F (1976) Biomechanics of the normal and diseased hip. An atlas. Springer, Berlin Heidel-berg New York

Pfeiffer KM, Meine J, Linder P (1975) Radiusfrakturen loco classico. Ther Umsch 32:788–799

Pfiffner A (1971) Die Daumensattelgelenksarthrose oder Rhizarthrose und Ergebnisse ihrer opera-tiven Behandlung. Arch Orthop Unfallchir 70:344–359

Pfitzner W (1892) Die Sesambeine des menschlichen Körpers. Morph Arb 1:517–762

Pieron A (1973) The mechanism of the first carpometacarpal (CMC) joint. Acta Orthop Scand [Suppl] 148:1–104

Ploetz E (1938) Funktioneller Bau und funktionelle Anpassung der Gleitsehne. Z Orthop 67: 212–234

Poigenfürst J, Tuchmann A (1978) Bedeutung der ulnaren Bandverletzung beim Speichenbruch an typischer Stelle. Handchirurgie 10:121–125

Poirier P, Charpy A (1911) Traité d'anatomie humaine, vol I. Masson, Paris

Preiser G (1908) Über pathologische Gelenkflächeninkongruenz. Zentralbl Chir 33:993–997

Ramselaar J (1970) Tendon transfer to restore opposition of the thumb. Stenfort Kroese, Leiden

Ray RD, Johnson RJ, Jameson RM (1951) Rotation of the forearm. An experimental study of pronation and supination. J Bone Joint Surg 33A:993–996

Reimann R, Ebner I (1980) Das menschliche Daumengrundgelenk – ein Eigelenk. Acta Anat (Basel) 108:1–9

Reinbach W-I (1952) Zur Entstehung der Membrana interossea antebrachii. Verh Anat Ges 50: 250–258

Rösli A (1963) Die Arthrographie, ein Beitrag zur Handgelenksdiagnostik. Schweiz Med Wochenschr 93:892–894

Rosenthal A (1949) Die Verletzungen des Discus articularis bei der typischen Radiusfraktur. Langenbecks Arch Chir 262:390–403

Rossak K (1965) Druckmessungen am Ellenbogengelenk. Verh Dtsch Orthop Ges 52:417–420

Rossak K (1970) Experimentelle Druckmessungen am Unterarm und ihre klinischen Folgen. Ergebn Chir Orthop 54:141–175

Roux W (1895) Gesammelte Abhandlungen über Entwicklungsmechanik der Organismen. Vol 1 and 2. Engelmann, Leipzig

Schlegel KF (1965) Die Arthrose des Daumensattelgelenks. Ther Ggw 104:761–769

Schleicher A, Tillmann B, Zilles K (1980) Quantitative analysis of X-ray images with a television image analyser. Microsc Acta 83:189–196

Schmidt H-M, Lieb B (1981) Die Articulatio carpometacarpea pollicis des Menschen: Größenmerkmale und Krümmungsprofile der Gelenkflächen. Verh Anat Ges 75:665–667

Schneider H (1959) Die Abnützungserkrankungen der Sehnen und ihre Therapie. Thieme, Stuttgart

Schneider PG (1964) Das Grazilissyndrom. Die Osteonecrosis pubica posttraumatica. Z Orthop 98:43–48

Segmüller G (1978) Das Mittelhandskelett in der Klinik. Huber, Bern

Shepherd F (1891) A note of the radio-carpal articulation. J Anat Physiol 25:349–351

Shiino K (1925) Einiges über die anatomischen Grundlagen der Greifbewegungen. Z Anat Entwicklungsgesch 77:344–357

Siegert F (1930) Das Problem des Metacarpale I und Metatarsale I. Z Anat Entwicklungsgesch 92:213–223

Sieglbauer F (1958) Lehrbuch der normalen Anatomie des Menschen, 8th edn. Urban and Schwarzenberg, München

Siegrist H (1980) Häufigere posttraumatische Beschwerden im Bereich der Hand. Rheumamedizin 2:121–128

Smith RJ (1974) Balance and kinetics of the fingers under normal and pathological conditions. J Clin Orthop Related Res 104:92–111

Spalteholz W (1896) Handatlas der Anatomie des Menschen. Sect I, Knochen, Gelenke, Bänder. Hirzel, Leipzig

Strasser H (1917) Lehrbuch der Muskel- und Gelenkmechanik, vol 4, Spezieller Teil. Die obere Extremität. Springer, Berlin

Stümpel E, Koebke J (in press) Zum funktionellen Bau der Fingergrundgelenke. Anat Anz

Swanson A (1972) Disabling arthritis at the base of the thumb (treatment by resection of the trapezium and flexible (silicone) implant arthroplasty). J Bone Joint Surg 54A:456–471

Swanson A (1980) Die Wiederherstellung der Daumensattelgelenke unter Berücksichtigung der Resektionsarthroplastik mit flexiblen Implantaten. Orthopaede 9:134–149

Taleisnik J (1976) The ligaments of the wrist. J Hand Surg 1:110–118

Tamega O, Machado de Sousa O, Bérzin F (1980) Analyse électromyographique du premier muscle interosseux dorsal de la main. I. Mouvements de l'index. Acta Anat (Basel) 107:214–220

Taylor G, Parsons CL (1938) The role of the discus articularis in Colles' fracture. J Bone Joint Surg 20:149–152

Testut L, Latarjet A (1948) Traité d'anatomie humaine, 9th edn. Doin, Paris

Thilenius G (1895) Das Os intermedium antebrachii des Menschen. Morph Arb 5:5–16

Thomas W (1977) Über die Ätiologie der Daumensattelgelenksarthrose und deren Behandlung durch eine spezielle Endoprothese. Z Orthop 115:699–707

Thomas W, Koebke J, Winter E (in press) Die Fibroostose an der Basis des Os metacarpale II und die Daumensattelgelenksarthrose. Orthop Prax

Thoms J (1962) Calcification of the triangular fibrocartilage in the wrist joint. Arthrographic study of a case. Br J Radiol 35:429–431

Tillmann B (1969) Die Beanspruchung des menschlichen Hüftgelenks. III. Die Form der Facies lunata. Z Anat Entwicklungsgesch 128:329–349

Tillmann B (1971) Die funktionelle Beanspruchung und Morphologie des menschlichen Ellenbogengelenks. Morph Jb 117:217–223

Tillmann B (1973) Zur Lokalisation von degenerativen Veränderungen am Femurkopf bei der Coxarthrose. Z Orthop 111:23–27

Tillmann B (1978) A contribution to the functional morphology of articular surfaces. Normale und pathologische Anatomie, vol 34. Thieme, Stuttgart

Tillmann B, Konermann H (1979) Zur "Tragfunktion" der Gelenkkapsel bei der Hüftluxation — Funktionelle und morphologische Untersuchungen. Orthop Prax 4:288–294

Tillmann K (1977) Überlegungen zur Pathogenese der Arthrose und ihre Bedeutung für die operative Therapie. Akt rheumatol 2:53–68

Tobler T (1929) Morphologische und histologische Befunde am Kniegelenkmeniskus in verschiedenen Lebensaltern. Schweiz Med Wochenschr 50:1359–1362

Toldt C (1911) Anatomischer Atlas 2. Lieferung C Bänderlehre, 7th edn. Urban and Schwarzenberg, Berlin

Vital JM, Lavignolle B, Sanchis G, Yates M, Constant P, Piton J, Sénégas J (1980) A study of the two forearm bones during pronation and supination movements in living subjects. Anat Clin 2:57–64

Von Baeyer H (1930) Der lebendige Arm. Fischer, Jena

Von Bardeleben K (1906) Lehrbuch der systematischen Anatomie des Menschen, Sect. I. Urban and Schwarzenberg, Berlin

Von Langer C, Toldt C (1911) Lehrbuch der systematischen und topographischen Anatomie, 9th edn. Braumüller, Wien

Von Lanz T, Wachsmuth W (1959) Praktische Anatomie, vol I, pt 3, Arm. 3rd edn. Springer, Berlin Göttingen Heidelberg

Waldeyer A (1950) Anatomie des Menschen. Pt 2, Kopf und Hals, Sehorgan, Ohr, Gehirn, obere Gliedmaße, Brust. de Gruyter, Berlin

Weidenreich F (1923) Knochenstudien. II. Teil: Über Sehnenverknöcherungen und Faktoren der Knochenbildung. Z Anat Entwicklungsgesch 69:558–597

Weissman JA, Legsdinsch AJ (1979) Das röntgenologische Bild des normalen Handgelenkraumes. Fortschr Röntgenstr 131:428–433

Wood Jones F (1944) The principles of anatomy as seen in the hand. 2nd edn. Bailliere, London

Zrubecky G (1960) Die Hand. Das Tastorgan des Menschen. Z Orthop 93:Beilageheft

Subject Index

Adduction
- thumb 32, 50
- ulna 29

Adductive malposition 50, 72
Arthrography 7, 19, 20
- method 3

Arthrosis
- metacarpophalangeal joints 57, 58, 68, 72
- proximal wrist joint 7, 27, 28
- saddle joint 33, 45, 53, 54, 72

Bone density 56, 61
- sclerosis 36
- spur 34, 50, 51
- subchondral 36, 60, 66

Cartilage
- cells 24, 61, 62
- degeneration 12, 36, 45, 50, 57
- localization 9, 12, 36, 45
- tangential fiber layer 47
- thickness 12, 66

Causal histogenesis 24, 52
Chondrocytes 11, 61
Collagen fibers 11, 12
Collateral ligaments
- metacarpophalangeal joints 49, 54, 61, 63
- proximal wrist joint 3, 4

Congruency 25, 33

Density measurements 40, 56
Disk
- anchorage 8, 12, 22, 26
- degeneration 2, 7, 21
- histology 11, 23
- perforation 2, 21, 25

Equidenses 40, 56, 62

Fracture experiments 15, 18, 27
- radius 3, 6, 26, 31
- styloid process 18, 26

Grip
- power 66, 68
- precision 66, 68

Hydrostatic point 24
- pressure 23

Incongruency 27, 33, 45, 49

Interosseous membrane 2, 3, 13, 29, 30
Isochromes 34, 39
Isoclines 56, 66

Joint capsule
- connections 7, 19
- contact 33, 39, 45, 72
- proximal wrist joint 19, 31
- saddle joint 33, 49
- stress 39, 47, 50

Kinetic energy 13, 15
- measurement 4, 6, 29

Loose body 34, 41, 53

Membrane see interosseous membrane
Metacarpophalangeal joints
- movements 54, 55, 64, 73

Opposition 31, 43, 55
Os lunatum 12, 25
- metacarpale I 32, 50, 55
- metarcarpale II 36, 44
- scaphoideum 18
- trapezium 43, 44, 47, 50
- triquetrum 22

Pisiform joint 7
Photoelastic experiments
- methods 34, 56, 73
- models 34, 37, 56, 69
Polarized light 34, 56
Pronation 13, 25, 29

Radius
- fracture 3, 6, 22, 25
Roentgenograms 3, 4, 33
Rotation 32, 44, 47, 53, 62

Saddle joint
- capsule 33, 49, 50
- ligaments 33, 49, 50
Singular point
- attractive 7, 9, 23, 37, 48
- repulsive 7, 37, 48
Split lines
- documentation 4, 56
- interpretation 23, 48, 68
- production 4, 56
Subluxation 26, 34, 50
Supination 13, 29
Strain gauges 4, 6

Advances in Anatomy Embryology and Cell Biology

Editors: F. Beck, W. Hild,
J. van Limborgh, R. Ortmann,
J.E. Pauly, T.H. Schiebler

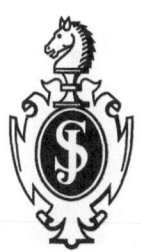

Springer-Verlag
Berlin
Heidelberg
New York
Tokyo

Volume 71: L. Thuneberg
Interstitial Cells of Cajal: Intestinal Pacemaker Cells?
1982. 94 figures. VII, 130 pages. ISBN 3-540-11261-8

Volume 72: H. Breuker
Seasonal Spermatogenesis in the Mute Swan (Cygnus olor)
1982. 30 figures. VII, 94 pages. ISBN 3-540-11326-6

Volume 73: G. Zweers
The Feeding System of the Pigeon (Columba livia L.)
1982. 45 figures. VII, 108 pages. ISBN 3-540-11332-0

Volume 74: J. Altman, S.A. Bayer
Development of the Cranial Nerve Ganglia and Related Nuclei in the Rat
1982. 64 figures. VII, 90 pages. ISBN 3-540-11337-1

Volume 75: V. Grouls, B. Helpap
The Development of the Red Pulp in the Spleen
1982. 37 figues. 80 pages. ISBN 3-540-11408-4

Volume 76: P. Kugler
On Angiotensin-Degrading Aminopeptidases in the Rat Kidney
1982. 88 figures. 96 pages. ISBN 3-540-11452-1

Volume 77. E. Braak
On the Structure of the Human Striate Area
1982. 44 figures. XI, 87 pages. ISBN 3-540-11512-9

Volume 78: G. Grün
The Development of the Vertebrate Retina: A Comparative Survey
1982. 15 figures. VIII, 85 pages. ISBN 3-540-11770-9

Volume 79: S.F. Perry
Reptilian Lungs
Functional Anatomy and Evolution
1983. 32 figures. Approx. 80 pages. ISBN 3-540-12194-3

J. Guyot

Atlas of
Human Limb Joints

Illustrations by J. L. Vannson
Translated from the French by R. A. Elson
1981. 113 figures. X, 252 pages
ISBN 3-540-10380-5

Contents: The Hip Joint. – The Knee Joint. – The Joints of the Foot. – The Shoulder Girdle and Shoulder Joints. – The Elbow Joint. – The Wrist Joint. – The Joints of the Hand. – References. – International Anatomical Nomenclature. – Subject Index.

Theoretical accounts of human anatomy have up to now lacked a practical demonstration of the functional activity in limb joints. In this book, the author closes this gap to provide the most complete description of human limb joints available today. The over 100 meticulously prepared drawings, diagrams and photographs illustrating the limb joints and their surrounding ligamentous structures are supplemented by a concise summary of functional anatomy. The careful attention to detail which the author and his colleagues have lavished upon this work will make it an indispensable reference for anatomists, radiologists, orthopedic surgeons, rheumatologists, and physicians active in the field of joint pathology, as well as for physical therapists, sports doctors, masseurs and medical students.

F. Pauwels

Biomechanics of the
Locomotor Apparatus

Contributions on the Functional Anatomy of the Locomotor Apparatus

Translated from the German, completely revised and enlarged, including seven new chapters

Translated by P. Maquet, R. Furlong

1980. 733 figures, 22 tables. VIII, 518 pages
ISBN 3-540-09131-9
Distribution rights for Japan: Nankodo, Tokyo

This classical work of functional anatomy results from more than forty years of study of the adaptation of the human locomotor apparatus to its specific functions.
These concepts revolutionize the theories previously accepted. Moreover, the author describes how to modify the stresses arising in the tissues in order to achieve therapeutic effects. In this way, he has the first to give a logical solution to the problem of the fractured neck of femur.
The concepts of Pauwels are clear. They are confirmed by clinical examples and by histological, anatomical and pathological preparations. They provide the basis for a logical anad scientific approach to orthopedic surgery.

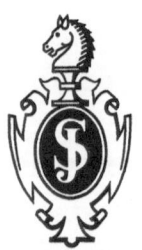

Springer-Verlag
Berlin
Heidelberg
New York
Tokyo

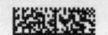